ADHD

Help Your Kids Reach Their Full Potential and Become Self-Regulated, Focused, and Confident

BILL ANDREWS

ANIVYA PUBLISHING

© Copyright 2019 - All rights reserved.

The content contained within this book may not be reproduced, duplicated or transmitted without direct written permission from the author or the publisher.

Under no circumstances will any blame or legal responsibility be held against the publisher, or author, for any damages, reparation, or monetary loss due to the information contained within this book. Either directly or indirectly.
Legal Notice:

This book is copyright protected. This book is only for personal use. You cannot amend, distribute, sell, use, quote or paraphrase any part, or the content within this book, without the consent of the author or publisher.
Disclaimer Notice:

Please note the information contained within this document is for educational and entertainment purposes only. All effort has been executed to present accurate, up to date, and reliable, complete information. No warranties of any kind are declared or implied. Readers acknowledge that the author is not engaging in the rendering of legal, financial, medical or professional advice. The content within this book has been derived from various sources. Please consult a licensed professional before attempting any techniques outlined in this book.
By reading this document, the reader agrees that under no circumstances is the author responsible for any losses, direct or indirect, which are incurred as a result of the use of information contained within this document, including, but not limited to, — errors, omissions, or inaccuracies.

CONTENTS

	Introduction	1
1	Understanding ADHD	3
2	ADHD Symptoms and Associated Conditions	13
3	The Impact of ADHD at School	27
4	When and How to Seek a Professional Diagnosis of ADHD	43
5	Treating ADHD	53
6	Therapy and Counseling as an ADHD Treatment	63
7	Methods for Living with an ADHD Child	75
8	Looking on the Bright Side of ADHD	87
9	Conclusion	97

INTRODUCTION

ADHD affects millions of children's lives every day. It also impacts the lives of parents and families. Understanding ADHD can be hard for even the most educated minds, but understanding is where treatment and management begins. While treatments for ADHD have come leaps and bounds compared to 20 years ago, there is still no single proven way to ensure successful treatment and management of ADHD. Fortunately, there are numerous options available to assist you in helping your child live his very best life.

The following chapters will discuss all aspects of ADHD in depth. You will start by gaining a full understanding of exactly what ADHD is, along with explanations of the different types of ADHD and its possible causes. The symptoms of ADHD will be explained in detail, so you will know what to look for and when. You will also gain great insight into the impact of ADHD on your entire family, as well as its impact at school and on your child's education. Since obtaining a medical diagnosis is paramount to treating ADHD, you will also learn step-by-step instructions for getting a professional diagnosis for your child.

In addition to learning all of this invaluable information that will help you understand ADHD, you will also find information in this book discussing the various treatment options available to your child. There is often much debate over using prescription medications to treat ADHD in children, so medications will be thoroughly discussed, as will alternative methods of treating ADHD without prescriptions. You will learn about the benefits of therapy for the entire family unit and even some potential disadvantages of a therapy. Finally, you will get the chance to learn hands-on methods of living with an ADHD child and managing behaviors at home. Suggestions for discipline and ideas for activities to keep your child busy are also included.

Completing your journey of ADHD education, you will discover a remarkable method of finding the bright side of ADHD and how your child can absolutely live a normal life. ADHD is not an ending—it is merely a new beginning of the next chapter of your child's life!

There are plenty of books on this subject on the market, thanks again for choosing this one! Every effort was made to ensure it is full of as much useful information as possible, please enjoy!

CHAPTER 1:

UNDERSTANDING ADHD

ADHD—everyone has heard about it or thought about it at some point in their lives. They may even know someone who has been diagnosed with ADHD. However, it is doubtful that the average person truly understands ADHD and its effect not only on the individual but also on the family unit. There are still plenty of "old school" folks who feel that ADHD is simply a made-up condition to excuse a lack of old-fashioned discipline. These people like to say how there was not any ADHD "back in their day." It is essential to remember that this is no longer 1972, and ADHD is an actual medical disorder that affects both children and adults today.

WHAT IS ADHD?

The first step in understanding ADHD is to fully comprehend exactly what it is. This is more than just a simple definition, although you will learn the definition of ADHD. Understanding exactly what ADHD really is includes learning about it from every aspect including but not limited to different types of ADHD and its possible causes. As a parent, knowing all that you can possibly know about the disorder will only aid you in providing the best environment for your ADHD child.

In the past, you may have heard the term ADD, also known as Attention Deficit Disorder. ADHD is an acronym for Attention-Deficit and Hyperactivity Disorder. ADD used to be considered a different condition than ADHD because it did not include hyperactivity. However, ADD is now considered to be an obsolete term, one that is no longer recognized by the American Psychiatric Association. Instead, the diagnosis, ADHD is used to describe disorders involving attention deficits.

ADHD is defined as a continuing neurobehavioral disorder that is characterized by inattentive, hyperactive, and/or impulsive behaviors. While most often diagnosed during the childhood years, many adults are also diagnosed with ADHD after reaching adulthood. While occasional inattentive, hyperactive, and impulsive behaviors are normal in all children and even in adults, these behaviors in combination with each other and other symptoms are no longer chalked up to a simple lack of discipline or self-control, or kids just being kids. ADHD is a recognized medical disorder that is estimated to affect approximately 17 million adults and children in the United States. It is believed that roughly 1 in 20 children have ADHD.

When it comes to understanding ADHD, remember that an ADHD diagnosis is not just an uncomplicated, one-size-fits-all medical finding. In fact, there are three distinct sub-types of ADHD described below with a few notable behavioral symptoms.

- **Predominantly Inattentive ADHD**: This sub-type of ADHD used to be referred to as ADD. Common behavioral symptoms include being disorganized, struggling to focus, and being forgetful. Notice that this sub-type of ADHD presents no signs of being hyperactive.

- **Predominantly Hyperactive-Impulsive ADHD**: This sub-type of ADHD includes behavioral symptoms of restlessness, such as constantly fidgeting and talking excessively. Impulsive behavioral symptoms are also noted. For example, interrupting conversations and not waiting for their turn. Most notably, this sub-type of ADHD does not include inattention. Children with this sub-type are able to focus on things that hold their interest—sometimes to the point of hyper-focusing.

- **Combined ADHD**: The third sub-type of ADHD, combined ADHD, is simply a combination of both predominantly inattentive and predominantly hyperactive-impulsive

ADHD. Behavioral symptoms include impulsivity, inattention, and hyperactivity.

Adult ADHD symptoms are not the same as ADHD symptoms in a child. In adults, inattention can include lacking motivation, forgetting to do day-to-day tasks, such as taking out the trash and losing things like car keys and important documents. Hyperactivity in adults may mean changing jobs frequently, feeling restless all the time, and not completing projects or tasks because of boredom. Impulsive behaviors in adults might involve being reckless with self-health, such as having unprotected sex with multiple partners and driving recklessly. Adults with ADHD may also find it hard to resist spending money and they may get called out for "not having a filter," which is speaking before thinking about what they are saying.

WHAT CAUSES ADHD?

As with any other medical diagnosis, the first thing a person wants to know is what caused the problem—in this case, ADHD. While it may be easier to believe that ADHD is caused by vaccines or even the overconsumption of sugar, there is no substantial scientific evidence to support those beliefs. The first thing to remember is that ADHD is a neurobiological disorder. Neurobiology is a life science that studies the cells of the nervous system and how these cells form circuits that not only process information but also regulate behavior. Since all types of ADHD deal with behavioral issues, it is easier to see how neurobiology and ADHD go hand in hand.

There is no single, underlying cause of ADHD. You are not going to find a magical answer in this book, one that will finally explain why your child struggles with ADHD. It is often a combination of factors, both neurobiological and environmental, that lead to the development of ADHD. Images of the brains of both ADHD children and non-ADHD children have revealed some interesting facts. While the brain development of both is quite similar, children with ADHD have a developmental delay of approximately 3 years in certain parts of the brain that are related to executive functions.

Executive functions are processes within the brain that deal with self-management. These functions include emotional and impulse control, flexible thinking that allows for the unexpected, a working memory that holds onto information, and the ability to plan and solve problems. A developmental delay in these executive functions means that ADHD children often act as many as three years younger than their peers. In other words, your ADHD child may seem much more immature than his playmates of the same age.

Studies have also indicated that there are other variances between the brains of an ADHD child and a non-ADHD child. There are notable differences in the chemical activity of the brain when it is communicating within itself. This means that when one part of the brain is telling another part of the brain what to do, the chemical activity varies in an ADHD child compared to a non-ADHD child. Research has also revealed that the parts of the brain that control attention have lower levels of activity in an ADHD child.

There are different potential environmental causes for ADHD. A child that is exposed to nicotine and/or alcohol has a higher chance of developing ADHD. A child that is born prematurely also has an increased risk for ADHD. It is additionally believed that a truly significant head injury can result in the development of ADHD. This is more likely to happen when the executive function areas of the brain are damaged due to the injury. In rare instances, it has been shown that exposure to environmental toxins may lead to the development of ADHD. One toxin is lead, which has been shown to interfere with a child's development and behavior after prolonged exposure. While there are clearly potential environmental factors that might cause ADHD, there is no definite factor or factors that lead to it—only environmental factors that may contribute to its development.

One other component that can increase a child's chance of developing ADHD is simple genetics. If there is a history of ADHD in a child's family, that child is more likely to develop ADHD. Statistically, there is a 25% chance that one parent of an ADHD child also has ADHD, even if the parent is not aware. Between genetics, the inner functioning of the brain, and environmental factors, there truly is not one absolute cause of ADHD. Realizing this, parents often feel some type of relief knowing that they are not solely to blame for their child's disorder.

HOW ADHD AFFECTS THE FAMILY UNIT

ADHD can have a profound effect on the life of the diagnosed child from childhood through adulthood. ADHD is not always something that a person eventually outgrows. It is a neurobiological disorder that has about a 50% chance of being a part of a person's life indefinitely. While the symptoms can be treated, the condition is not guaranteed to disappear. ADHD not only affects the child, it also affects the family of the child. After all, one person in the family unit now has a medical disorder that affects the child's behavior. Behavioral symptoms can be quite difficult to cope with on a daily basis for everyone in the family from parents to siblings. Even extended family members can be affected by the diagnosis, such as a grandparent or aunt/uncle that babysits the ADHD child. Here, we will discuss how ADHD can affect the families of toddlers, prepubescent children, teenagers, and adults.

ADHD Toddlers and Families: Toddlers are known for being impulsive, extremely active, and lacking a long attention span. These common occurrences can make it difficult to determine if a toddler has ADHD. If a toddler is diagnosed with ADHD, the diagnosis is likely to affect the entire family. An ADHD toddler requires immense supervision compared to a non-ADHD toddler. Of course, all toddlers need plenty of supervision, however, when a parent is dealing with an ADHD toddler, it requires a different parenting approach. An ADHD toddler may not respond to a parent's directions and commands the way that a non-ADHD toddler responds. This can lead to a parent suffering from feelings of inadequacy or failure as a parent. It can also increase the amount of stress on parents. As if it is not difficult enough to take care of a toddler, throwing ADHD into the mix does nothing to help.

ADHD Prepubescent Children and Families: Even as a child grows older, the demands on the family do not stop. A preadolescent child with ADHD is likely to exhibit even more behavioral symptoms of the condition. The child may act out more than the average child. The impulsiveness associated with the condition may manifest itself with the child struggling to behave. This is often when parents begin to notice that ADHD is affecting the child's education. Parents and teachers must work together to discuss the behaviors, form a plan to address the behaviors, and present a united front to the child. Since the ADHD child is now spending a good part of the day with his peers, the parents may notice that the child does not have many friends or is not invited to play dates and birthday parties. This is often the result of the ADHD behaviors disrupting social settings. Other parents simply may not have the patience or the desire to handle an ADHD child in their home.

Older ADHD children may struggle with getting a good night's sleep. ADHD children usually do not require as much sleep as other kids. Their bodies are able to function on little sleep because of the hyperactivity associated with ADHD. However, just because these children can function on little sleep does not mean that they do not need sleep. Sleep is the body's way of shutting down, relaxing, and re-energizing for the next day. Sleep is healing for the body and the brain. Lack of sleep can cause daytime behaviors to become even more prominent. Imagine how grumpy an adult can be without a good night's sleep. Now, think about how an ADHD child must feel without restful sleep. They are practically running on adrenaline. The lack of sleep will also affect the family, either by the child waking up siblings or the parents having to wake up to put the child back to bed.

Again, this adds more stress and pressure to the family unit. The ADHD child, regardless of age, requires constant supervision. Other siblings in the family may feel that the ADHD child gets the most attention. Siblings may grow resentful of the attention being taken away from them. There may also be increased arguments between the ADHD child and his siblings. As parents have to constantly play referee, their stress levels rise. Again, feelings of inadequacy or failure may start to set in. Stress and tension in a family unit are often picked up on by the ADHD child and non-ADHD siblings. This only increases the stress and frustration felt by all.

Older ADHD children may exhibit additional aggressive behaviors, such as physical fighting with siblings. Since parenting an ADHD child requires a more patient approach, siblings may feel as if they are being punished for the behavior of the ADHD child. For instance, a physical fight between an 8-year-old ADHD child and a 10-year-old sibling will likely find both children being disciplined. However, the 10-year-old sibling may feel that the ADHD sibling started the fight, and they were only defending themselves. Once more, siblings are left feeling that they are not as special or as important as the ADHD child, or the ADHD child gets away with behaviors and is the favored child. Parents are left to figure out how to discipline fairly while keeping the condition in mind.

ADHD Teens and Families: Going through puberty and becoming a teen is difficult for all children. The changes in the body and the hormone levels are hard to handle even without adding in ADHD. The ADHD teen faces an entirely new set of challenges. The family unit faces new challenges, as well. No longer are the parents tending to a rowdy toddler or rambunctious child. They are now faced with a young adult who is simply trying to find his way in the world and figure out exactly who he is—all while coping with the symptoms of ADHD.

ADHD teens may be even more aggressive than their younger selves. Parents may also notice that their teen has become antisocial. The average teen goes through so many ups and downs as they become adults, both physically and emotionally, that a quiet, sullen teenager normally is not something to worry about. However, if that teen has been diagnosed with ADHD, parents must be even more vigilant. ADHD teens can be prone to breaking the rules, breaking the law, and taking risks with their lives. These behaviors are a result of the lack of impulse control. Simply put, ADHD teens have trouble thinking about the consequences of their actions. They are more focused on the here and now, on the instant gratification.

The family unit still struggles even during the teen years. A younger child might have temper tantrums, but he is still young and seeking parental approval. That means that the younger ADHD child is more likely to get over whatever set him off and talk it out with the family. An ADHD teen, however, will often keep things bottled up inside, much like the non-ADHD teen. This becomes a time when communication is extremely important between the ADHD teen, parents, siblings, and other affected family members. This is also an important period for communication with the child's teachers. ADHD teens have a higher chance of academic failure. Just as when the child was younger, parents and teachers have to form an alliance to ensure that the teen stays on track academically.

ADHD Adults and Families: ADHD does not stop affecting the entire family just because a child reaches adulthood. Instead, ADHD just becomes a problem for the adult. The ADHD adult may find it hard to stay at one job. It is not because he does not like the job—it is only because he grows bored quickly and needs a change to keep him interested. Married ADHD adults may find that it is a struggle to give their family the structure and stability they require and deserve. It can be easy for the ADHD mom to get angry quickly with her children if they are bothering her while she is focused on another task. An adult ADHD short fuse is different than the agitation of a non-ADHD adult. The anger can quickly escalate out of control, resulting in hateful words and hurt feelings. If the ADHD parent spends money on a whim, this can lead to a financial burden on the family, especially the non-ADHD spouse. Procrastination and disorganization are prevalent in an ADHD adult. While these behaviors are not such a big deal when the adult is single, they can become quite bothersome in a family unit. Schedules are necessary for families, and a clean and organized home simply makes life easier. With an ADHD adult in the family, it is not uncommon for schedules and organization to go right out the window.

One of the biggest issues affecting the family unit because of ADHD is marital problems. No, the ADHD child does not cause the problems in the marriage. Rather, the added stress and tension of living with and dealing with the disorder can lead to marital issues. Perhaps the financial cost of seeking treatment for the disorder has put a strain on the family finances. Maybe the disruptive behavior leads to arguments between the parents on discipline matters. Regardless of the age of the ADHD child, parents must remember that it is not the child's fault—he did not ask for the disorder. Instead of falling apart as a married couple, the parents need to find common ground on which they can come together.

ADHD is not a disorder that affects only one person. It is a family condition, one that requires patience and perseverance to cope with every day. Often, family therapy is a good treatment option to help each member of the family learn how to deal with different behaviors. Family therapy also gives each person the chance to voice their feelings in a private and safe setting. ADHD does not have to be the end of a family. Yes, it will affect every family member. ADHD is not picky. It does not care what race or gender a person might be. It does not care if a person is rich or poor. However, ADHD affects the lives of millions of people around the entire world. Yet, these millions of people still manage to live regular lives and function as an individual and a family every day. Families must arm themselves with knowledge and commitment in order to sustain a happy, healthy home.

CHAPTER 2:

ADHD SYMPTOMS AND ASSOCIATED CONDITIONS

Now that you have a better understanding of exactly what ADHD is, its possible causes, and how ADHD can affect the entire family unit, it is time to delve deeper into the particular symptoms of each sub-type of ADHD. The symptoms are not always the same with each child, and the symptoms can vary depending on the age of the child. We will also take a closer look at other associated conditions that could also affect an ADHD child. Understanding and recognizing the possible symptoms of ADHD is necessary when you are trying to decide if your child's behaviors are normal or if they need further evaluation by a medical professional.

SYMPTOMS OF ADHD SUB-TYPES AND AGE GROUPS

As previously discussed, ADHD has three sub-types: Predominantly Inattentive ADHD, Predominantly Hyperactive-Impulsive ADHD, and Combined ADHD. Each sub-type has some of the same symptoms, as well as different symptoms associated with that particular sub-type. Recognizing possible ADHD symptoms is a vital step to understanding what your child is feeling and experiencing. After all, you cannot possibly know what is going on inside your child's head unless you also have ADHD. By understanding the symptoms, you will find it a little easier to be compassionate when needed. You may also find it easier to work out a plan for discipline since an ADHD child often does not respond to traditional disciplinary methods. Recognizing symptoms is likewise an essential step towards seeking a possible medical diagnosis, which is necessary for some treatment methods, as well as school-related adjustments to your child's learning plan. Here, we will take a closer look at each sub-type and their associated symptoms. We will then put these symptoms into perspective according to the different age groups of the affected children.

Predominantly Inattentive ADHD: This sub-type of ADHD was once identified as ADD because it lacks the symptom of hyperactivity. However, since the American Psychiatric Association no longer recognizes ADD as a disorder of its own, it has become known as a sub-type of general ADHD. There are various symptoms associated with Predominantly Inattentive ADHD. You may notice that it does not take much for your child to get distracted from one activity to another. He might also struggle to organize a particular project or task, such as laying out puzzle pieces or assembling a Lego toy. Your child may also be described as a daydreamer because he loses focus as his mind wanders off to other things.

A child with this sub-type of ADHD may struggle to follow precise directions, and it may even appear that your child is just simply not listening. You may also notice that your child is always losing things, such as pencils for homework or misplaced shoes on a regular basis. He may try to avoid chores and/or school work because they do not hold his interest. If you find yourself repeatedly reminding your child to finish his homework or take out the trash, it may turn into a constant battle if your child has this sub-type of ADHD. Your child's teachers may notice that he consistently makes careless mistakes in his school work. This often occurs because he has lost interest in the work, or he is in a hurry to finish because something else has caught his attention. If you notice that your child struggles to stay focused on the task at hand and this occurs regularly, it may be time to consider the possibility of ADHD.

Predominantly Hyperactive-Impulsive ADHD: This sub-type of ADHD differs from Predominantly Inattentive ADHD because a child with this disorder is able to pay attention. He may even stay focused on a task that holds his interest to the point that he blocks everything else around him out. A child with Hyperactive-Impulsive ADHD may be the talker of the family or in class. You may see that your child always has plenty to say about any subject being discussed, and he will often be in such a rush to speak that he repeatedly interrupts the conversation. In school, your child may talk without asking permission, or he may be known as the "class clown" because he is always up to something and trying to make his classmates laugh. He may blurt out answers to questions without permission from the teacher, simply because he cannot contain himself.

You may also observe a lot of movement from this form of ADHD child. If you find yourself describing your child as "always on the go," he may have this sub-type of ADHD. Your child may struggle to be still when it is required. For instance, his teacher may notice that he constantly fidgets and moves about at his desk. In church, you may see your child shifting positions, squirming, and really struggling to sit still. During playtime, your child will be quite active, even more than the average child. He may do a lot of physical activities, such as running, jumping, roughhousing, and climbing, even if these activities are not allowed at certain times. Your child may also be quite loud and boisterous with other children, to the point of disturbing others around him or even causing a scene.

The Predominantly Hyperactive-Impulsive ADHD child lacks impulse control. This means that he tends not to think before acting. He does not consider the consequences of his actions before he proceeds. This can be both a minor and a significant symptom. If your child talks out of turn or has difficulty waiting his turn for an activity, it could be related to a lack of impulse control. Those are minor instances. A significant instance might be your child putting himself in danger without being aware of it. For example, if your child chases a ball into the street without watching for cars, or if he takes daredevil risks riding his bike, he may be struggling to control his impulses. In other words, your child has a desire to do something, even if it is considered dangerous, but he feels invincible and does not consider the bad things that could happen.

Combined ADHD: The third sub-type of ADHD is Combined ADHD. This sub-type is a combination of both Predominantly Inattentive and Hyperactive-Impulsive ADHD. A child with combined ADHD will exhibit signs of both of the other sub-types. Basically, your child has drawn the shortest straw. Your child will have to deal with disorganization, lack of focus, daydreaming, constantly misplacing items, and following directions. He will also grapple with impulse control causing him to speak out of turn and struggle waiting for his turn. Patience is most definitely not your child's strong point. It may also lead him to take unsafe risks during activities and playtime. Your child is likely to be noisy and extremely active, always looking for something new to do but being easily distracted from each activity. The combined ADHD child is going to fidget and squirm because sitting still simply is not something his mind can demand from his body—at least not for extended periods of time.

This particular ADHD sub-type is the disorder that most people think of when they hear the term ADHD. They automatically picture a child with little to no self-control that cannot sit still, is aggressive, talks too much, does not complete school work or chores, and is just an overall difficult child. It is unfortunate that the average person views an ADHD child in this manner because ADHD, no matter which sub-type you are dealing with, is only a medical condition. It does not mean that the child is a hopeless cause. Children with ADHD should not be singled out for their disorder or looked at differently than their peers. Instead, adults need to be more sympathetic and understanding of the disorder.

ADHD Symptoms as Related to Age: Recognizing the symptoms of ADHD in your child may be easier to grasp if you look at it from the perspective of age. ADHD children of different age groups exhibit different symptoms of the disorder. For example, a teenager is not likely to bounce off the walls with excitement at the prospect of playing on the jungle gym the way that a 4th grader might react. Here, we will take a closer look at the different age/grade groups of ADHD children.

- **Toddlers:** Children that are 3 years of age and younger, or otherwise too young for school, are considered to be toddlers. Recognizing ADHD symptoms in toddlers is a challenging task. This is because toddlers are notoriously self-centered, easily agitated, and easily bored. It can be hard to know if your toddler jumps around from toy to toy because he is simply soaking in the new knowledge from each toy, or it is because his little brain lacks the ability to stay focused and pay attention to a particular toy. At this age, parents should take note of behaviors that seem repetitive, such as the toddler being unable to stay focused on an everyday basis, rather than just occasionally. It can be quite difficult to diagnose a toddler. ADHD symptoms are usually much easier to recognize with increased age.

- **Pre-Kindergarten through 2nd Grade:** Children that fall into this grade category normally range in ages from 4 to 7–8 years old. These children are still quite young, and they are still learning their limits and boundaries in supervised environments, both at home and at school. Your child may struggle to follow simple directions, or he may just ignore the directions outright so he can do things the way he wants to do them. An ADHD child at this age struggles with impulse and self-control. He may touch and/or hold items that he has been told to leave alone. Your child is probably in constant motion, whether it be fidgeting or wandering around the classroom when he is bored. You may also notice that getting your child to pay attention and listen is next to impossible. He has a lot of thoughts going through his mind at once so staying engaged is a problem. He is also likely to speak out of turn because he just cannot help himself.

- **3rd Grade through 8th Grade:** Children in this range of grades are usually ages 8 to 13–14 years old. There are numerous symptoms that you or your child's teacher may notice. Constant fidgeting and trying to sit still is a possible indicator. This continuous movement goes beyond the occasional squirminess of a young child. Not only will your child fidget, but he may also get up out of his seat whenever he feels like it without permission. You may also note that your child is quite restless and bored, both at home and at school. He may have difficulty concentrating on school assignments or consistently forgets to turn them in. Your child may be thought of as a daydreamer because his mind wanders off, and he no longer pays attention to whatever is going on around him. Children this age with ADHD often do not think of outcomes. They want to do what they want to do, and they want to do it now. It is not until later when a parent or teacher is explaining the consequences that the child takes the time to think about what he did.

- **9th grade to 12th grade:** Children in this grade category are no longer really children, they are young adults. Their ages range from 14 to 17–18 years old. These are teenagers you are dealing with, and teens are never easy to handle—even those without ADHD. ADHD teens do not exhibit all of the symptoms that younger children display. The hyperactivity side of ADHD usually slows down as the child gets older. But it can manifest itself in other ways. For instance, instead of playing tag and running races with friends, your ADHD teen may find a task to focus on, such as artwork, and spend hours upon hours drawing or painting. You may also notice a total lack of organization in your ADHD teen. Your teen likely struggles with schedules and turning assignments in on time because he has trouble prioritizing things in his life. When assignments are turned in, they are often sloppy, full of mistakes, or obviously not completed.

Your ADHD teen is still going to be reckless. He will still have trouble thinking about his actions and the consequences before he does something. Unfortunately, with age, reckless behavior can start to pose a risk to the health and safety of your teenage child. He may take unnecessary risks while driving, such as speeding or even trying to text and drive at the same time. Your ADHD teen is still going to act upon impulse—he will get an idea and decide to pursue it without making a plan or thinking about what might happen. Planning is definitely not his strong suit. The ADHD teen prefers to act first and think later. This is an age when parents must be even more watchful than before because an ADHD teen could take chances with his safety.

With so many varying signs and symptoms of ADHD, it is no wonder that parents are easily confused when it comes to their own children. It is easy to question whether or not a behavior is normal or a cause for concern. The best thing parents can do is communicate with their child, as well as with other influential adults around their child, such as teachers or older siblings, and then they can decide if there is a pattern to the behaviors. It can be something as simple as taking notes in a journal on a day-to-day basis. Later, after a month or two, the parents can read through the journal, and they can decide if professional help is needed. As long as you are an aware and involved parent, if your child does exhibit signs of ADHD or another type of disorder, you are most likely to be the first one to notice.

ASSOCIATED CONDITIONS OF ADHD

As if a diagnosis of ADHD is not enough for a parent to worry about, there are often other conditions that develop in conjunction with ADHD or simply as a reaction to ADHD. Children with ADHD and an associated condition require that much more time, attention, and medical care. It is believed that approximately half of all people with ADHD also have another condition. In children, the Centers for Disease Control and Prevention estimates that approximately 2/3 of ADHD children have another disorder. Associated conditions can be mild or severe. They might be directly linked to ADHD, or they might be a condition that has simply taken its time to show up and announce its presence. These additional conditions fall within two categories: secondary conditions and comorbid conditions.

Secondary conditions are those that are a direct result of the ADHD. When a child is dealing with ADHD, it can be quite a frustrating and stressful situation for him. In many cases, other conditions develop because they are triggered by frustration and stress. As treatment of the ADHD progresses, these secondary conditions often become more manageable or fade away entirely. Comorbid conditions are conditions that exist concurrently with ADHD. They are not going away with the ADHD treatment. In fact, comorbid conditions usually need their own specific treatment program. It is essential that you and your child's doctor determine which additional conditions are secondary or comorbid.

The number of associated conditions a child or adult can have along with ADHD is basically endless. There simply is not enough time or book space to discuss every possible medical condition because they are not all definitively associated with ADHD. However, it is important to know some of the common conditions and their possible symptoms because when it comes to ADHD, knowledge is power. While not an all-inclusive list of probable related conditions, the following list describes many of the more prevalent associated conditions.

- **Anxiety** – We have all felt a little anxious at some point in our lives. Anxiety manifests itself as feelings of stress, worry, being tense, being tired, and several other symptoms. However, the fleeting anxiety the average person feels is not considered a disorder. Chronic anxiety affects about 30% of ADHD children and approximately 50% of ADHD adults. These feelings of worry and stress can have a detrimental effect on the quality of life. Depending on whether or not the anxiety begins to diminish with ADHD treatment determines if it is a secondary or comorbid condition.

- **Depression** – Depression is a mood disorder that affects almost 15% of ADHD children and almost 50% of ADHD adults. Only about 1% of non-ADHD children suffer from depression. Depression is more than a few moments of feeling sad. Everyone feels sad from time to time. Depression is a serious disorder that involves feeling unhappy, moody, irritable, and even worthless. These feelings do not go away. Depression affects more than just your mood—it reduces your interest in life. It requires treatment, often including therapy. Depression may occur because of ADHD or because of environmental factors and genetic predisposition. In most cases, it is considered a comorbid condition.

- **Learning and language disabilities** – As much as 50% of ADHD children have a type of learning disorder. When compared to only 5% of non-ADHD children having learning disorders, this number is quite compelling. Dyslexia and dyscalculia are two of the more common learning syndromes that may affect an ADHD child. Dyslexia has an impact on the child's ability to read and write. Dyscalculia impacts the child's ability to understand and perform math skills. Language disorders affect approximately 12% of ADHD children, while these speech problems only affect about 3% of non-ADHD children. Both learning and language disabilities fall into the category of comorbid conditions. They each require their own treatment plan.

- **Gross and fine motor skill difficulties** – Fine motor skills include tasks like grasping a pencil with your fingers and writing. Gross motor skills include physical activities, such as jumping and running. Both types of skills require the use of certain small or large sets of muscles. ADHD can affect the fine and gross motor skills of your child. For example, you may notice that your child struggles to write neatly because his hand and fingers jerk around. Your child may seem awkward and overly clumsy, such as falling frequently or struggling to do a jumping jack, because the ADHD is affecting larger sets of muscles. These disorders are comorbid conditions and require their own treatment plan.

- **Obsessive-compulsive disorder** – Obsessive-compulsive disorder also known as OCD, may have you thinking of the hoarding shows on television. While hoarding certainly is a symptom of OCD, it is not the only symptom. This disorder can be mild or extreme. It can manifest itself in the form of repetitive behavior, like counting to a certain number while performing a task, or even pulling out hair. OCD can also involve the extreme need to be clean, such as washing hands repeatedly, even until they are raw. OCD may involve hoarding, which is the overwhelming desire to collect certain items, or it can be a form of extreme anxiety to the point of being overly cautious. OCD is also a comorbid condition. Therapeutic treatment can be helpful, along with possible medications.

- **Oppositional defiant disorder** – Oppositional defiant disorder is a common disorder associated with ADHD and known as ODD. This disorder results in extreme bouts of anger and/or rage. This is not a typical temper tantrum. ODD is uncontrollable anger/rage that occurs during a meltdown that results from even the smallest trigger. These meltdowns can last just a few minutes or even as long as half an hour. When an ODD child has a meltdown, once he has calmed down, he is usually quite remorseful about what happened. This disorder can be secondary or comorbid. There are various types of treatment available.

- **Bipolar disorder** – Bipolar disorder is another mood disorder that has various symptoms. It is a comorbid disorder, so you cannot expect the ADHD treatment to fix the bipolar problem. Bipolar disorder often includes severe and unexplainable mood swings. For example, your child may be ecstatic and extremely happy for several days, only to suddenly switch gears to anger and rage that also lasts for several days. People with bipolar disorder have a hard time relaxing and calming down, especially when they are in a "manic" state of mind. There are numerous medical treatments to help control bipolar disorder because even though the "highs" feel great to the patient, the "lows" may feel worse than anything they have ever felt—possibly driving them to the point of suicide.

- **Tic disorder** – A tic disorder involves physical twitching of certain groups of muscles. These muscles are often found in the face, neck, and shoulder areas of the body. You may notice short, jerking movements of your child's head that he cannot stop or control. You may even detect tics of the eyes or the mouth, such as the rapid and uncontrolled blinking of the eyes or a chronic twitch at the corner of the mouth. Tics are most often noticed in children, and many children ultimately grow out of the tic disorder as they become an adult. It was once believed that certain stimulant ADHD medications caused tic disorders. However, more has been learned about these types of conditions, including the fact that there is a genetic factor to consider. It is now believed that the stimulant medications did not cause the tic disorder, the medication simply flipped on the internal, genetic predisposition switch residing within the child. Tic disorders are comorbid disorders and can be managed with appropriate treatment.

- **Tourette syndrome** – This is a syndrome that most people misunderstand. A person hears the word Tourette and they automatically assume that the afflicted will randomly blurt out swear words. This is not the movies—this is real life. It is also interesting to note that about 60-80% of people with this particular syndrome also have ADHD, but not even 10% of ADHD people have Tourette syndrome. Tourette syndrome does manifest itself in a vocal manner. Think of it like tics, only it is tics of the vocal cords. People with this disorder may make odd noises randomly or repeat phrases indiscriminately, including the occasional swear word. However, uncontrolled swearing is not a realistic description of Tourette syndrome. This is a comorbid condition that requires a different treatment plan than ADHD.

- **Sleep disorder** – It is extremely common for ADHD children to have struggles with sleep. They may have trouble falling asleep, they may have difficulty staying asleep, or they may have both problems. Sleeping disorders are often a secondary condition of ADHD. There are treatments available that can help your child to fall asleep and stay asleep. These treatments used in conjunction with the ADHD treatment plan should make for a happier, well-rested child.

- **Abuse of substances** – Studies have indicated that ADHD children have a higher risk of smoking cigarettes at an early age. They also have an added risk of following this nicotine dependence with alcohol abuse and, in severe cases, even drug abuse. ADHD children are twice as likely to develop an addiction to nicotine. It is important to note that studies show ADHD children treated with stimulant medications are less likely than their non-ADHD peers to abuse illegal stimulants, such as cocaine and methamphetamine. This may be a result of the opposite effect that stimulants have on ADHD children. These substance abuse problems are a secondary result of ADHD. In many cases, with the appropriate treatment, parents can be proactive and prevent substance abuse from ever becoming a problem by actively treating the ADHD.

Secondary and comorbid conditions include many more than this list defines. Your child could be suffering from any sort of condition at this very moment without your knowledge. That is why it is essential that parents are involved in their children's lives and keep the lines of communication open. Many of these associated conditions are serious and require their own form of treatment. If your child is diagnosed with ADHD, you cannot assume that the ADHD treatment plan is going to solve all of the problems, both behavioral and emotional. Instead, monitor your child and his reaction to the treatment plan. If you still notice obvious problems, even after tweaking the treatment plan, it may be time to consider the idea that your child has an associated condition.

Obviously, this list of potentially associated conditions is quite overwhelming and it is not an all-inclusive list. There are numerous other conditions that are not mentioned, which could be associated with ADHD. Parents must keep in mind that an ADHD diagnosis does not automatically equate a diagnosis of a second disorder. It is also important to note that some of these associated conditions can be mistaken for ADHD. This is why a medical examination, testing, and professional diagnosis are necessary. If you treat your child for ADHD when he is actually suffering from bipolar disorder or anxiety and depression, it can pose a serious threat to his overall health and well-being. Associated conditions are not necessarily the norm—there are millions of children and adults that cope with only ADHD on a daily basis. However, knowing about the possible associated conditions and recognizing some of the symptoms helps to ensure that your child's mental health is always at its best.

CHAPTER 3:

THE IMPACT OF ADHD AT SCHOOL

ADHD is not just a condition that affects the home life and family unit of the ADHD child. It affects every aspect of the child's life, including school, extracurricular activities, friendships, and family outings. One of the most significant areas that ADHD impacts is, not surprisingly, school. The education of your child is a very important part of your child's life. Education is vital in today's society. Even the most menial jobs require a minimum high school education. Complex careers like psychiatry or medicine require many more years of higher education and various degrees. Education is important for all children including your ADHD child. However, the impact of ADHD on your child's learning can pose a serious threat to your child's entire education.

School is not only supposed to give your child the knowledge he needs to pursue his dream career; it is also designed to teach your child many essential social skills. School is a place where kids interact with their peers. They begin to form friendships and bonds that could possibly last a lifetime. They learn how to behave in different social settings, such as at a basketball game or a school dance. They learn how to behave in classroom settings with specific rules and scheduling. From elementary school through high school, kids are learning new skills, gaining more knowledge, and they are immersed in group interactions. So, where and how does your ADHD child fit into all of this?

DIFFICULTIES ADHD PRESENTS IN A CLASSROOM SETTING

So far, we have learned that ADHD presents itself through a wide range of symptoms. These symptoms can include but are not limited to the following: daydreaming, lack of focus, not listening and paying attention, trouble following directions, hyperactivity, disruptive behavior, speaking out of turn, lack of impulse control, reckless behavior, aggression, irritability, constant fidgeting, disorganization, forgetfulness, loud, rambunctious, and so much more.

Now, think about a classroom setting. Does the classroom seem like the place where some or all of those characteristics might fit in? How many teachers do you know who allow disruptive and aggressive behaviors in class? School is a place with lots of rules and your ADHD child struggles to follow simple directions. How can he possibly succeed in school? What can you do to help him without hindering him? How can the teacher help? There are so many unanswered questions you probably have right now. Let's find the answers together.

ADHD is going to affect your child's time at school. It is as simple as that. Accepting this right off the bat is a good first step in helping your ADHD child succeed. Remember, just because the ADHD impacts your child's education does not necessarily mean that it is only going to have a negative result. ADHD kids go to school every day. You probably went to school with ADHD children. There are probably ADHD kids at school with your child right now. Just because a child has ADHD does not mean that it is always noticeable. After all, there are lots of treatment plans to explore. The bottom line is that your child can still be successful at school, even with ADHD.

Now that you have accepted that ADHD is, in fact, going to impact your child's classroom time, it is time to discuss some of the difficulties it may present. Your child may struggle with staying focused on classroom assignments. He is going to be easily distracted by the children around him or just by his own imagination. He may fail to complete classroom work and homework because it fails to capture his attention. He probably finds the whole classroom and learning setting quite boring. After all, there are so many more fun things he could be doing. Your ADHD child's inability to stay focused could result in poor grades—even possible failure.

Your ADHD child may also disrupt the class. He might fidget and squirm in his seat, making it impossible for him to concentrate on the lesson. This constant movement is going to disturb his classmates. He may even just get up out of his seat and wander around the classroom at times. This, of course, causes even more distraction among the rest of the students. There will be times when your ADHD child is simply bursting to talk, so he blurts out whatever he has to say without permission. He is going to interrupt the teacher with questions and comments. He is going to interrupt classmates in the same way. Your ADHD child will probably be one of the loudest kids in class. He may be the class clown because he does silly things for attention from his peers. Your ADHD child may have trouble with his temper. Being easily irritated could lead to shouting arguments or even physical fighting. There is a good possibility that ADHD is going to increase your child's chances of getting in trouble at school.

When your ADHD child is not talking out of turn and moving all around, he may be just the opposite. His teacher might notice that he seems to drift away frequently, caught up in his own daydreams. It will be obvious that he is not paying attention, not even hearing the words around him, because he is lost in his own thoughts and imaginings. Your ADHD child may need to be brought back to attention repeatedly, which can be quite disruptive to the entire class. His forgetfulness is not going to help him as far as keeping track of his school supplies and work. You will find yourself constantly reminding him to do his homework, gather his books, make sure he has enough paper and endless other reminders. ADHD often includes being unorganized. This mean folders and backpacks that are always a hot mess, notices from school that go undelivered to you because they were lost in the mess, and an overall intensification of stress for you and your child because nothing can ever be found right away.

All of these potential difficulties are going to add pressure to your already-stressed ADHD child. You, his teacher, and his classmates are also going to feel the effects. Stress levels will rise. There may be increased tensions between your child and his peers, as well as his teacher. Peers may feel that your child gets too much attention in class because the teacher has to stay on top of his behavior so much. Peers may feel that your ADHD child disrupts on purpose, which can lead to confrontation between your child and peers. Even the teacher is likely to feel frustration and stress from having to monitor your child so much when she has so many other responsibilities on her plate. So, what can you as the parent do to make things easier for everyone involved? The answer lies in teamwork.

TEAMWORK TO ADDRESS AND OVERCOME DIFFICULTIES

You, your ADHD child, and his teacher must work together as a team to face these potential difficulties. A united and supportive team is likely to make your child feel more secure with himself and the ADHD. Whether your child is in elementary school or high school, all involved parties must be on the same page working together to devise a daily ADHD plan. There are certain responsibilities that fall on your shoulders as the parent. There are also specific things the teacher can do at school. Your ADHD child must be a part of the plan. It takes teamwork between everyone to help your child succeed at school.

WORKING TOGETHER WITH THE TEACHER

The most important thing you can do is be honest with your child's teacher and school faculty. Do not try to hide the fact that he has ADHD. Not only will this make it impossible to work as a team to fit your child's needs, but it will also make your ADHD child feel ashamed and embarrassed about his disorder. Set up a private meeting with the teacher and the necessary faculty to inform them of his disorder and begin creating a plan. Rome was not built in a day, so expect many more meetings in the future.

At the first meeting, talk freely about your ADHD child's condition. Discuss his symptoms in detail, so his teacher will know what to expect on bad days. Discuss your child's medical history, including when ADHD was first diagnosed and how you approach treatment at home. Do not hold back. Your ADHD child's teacher and faculty team need full disclosure to assist them in creating a workable plan at school. Being completely truthful may be uncomfortable at times. No one enjoys talking about their child's difficulties, especially something like ADHD that can affect his behavior in so many negative ways. But withholding information will only delay your child's progress. Simply put, just be honest, and let it all out.

During the meetings, make sure you do not take personal offense to constructive criticism and advice. As mentioned, discussing your child's difficulties is not an easy task—not for any parent. Parents are notoriously protective of their children, and you are not an exception. But you cannot gloss over his ADHD. You cannot sugarcoat the symptoms and impact it has on his entire life. If advice is given, listen with an open mind and an open heart. The teacher is only trying to help the situation. If you develop an angry or dismissive attitude, communication will simply falter, and nothing substantial will be accomplished. Communication in a respectful manner is paramount to creating a successful education plan for school. Remember that you need your child's teacher on his team. Go in with an open mind, and come out with a solid plan.

Do not withhold vital information from your ADHD child's teacher. If he is taking prescription medication, the school needs to know. If he has an associated condition, it is imperative that you inform the school. The more details you can give his teacher, the better the plan you will construct together. Like we discussed earlier, this is a time for complete transparency. Your child's teacher and the involved faculty need the details—even the not-so-pretty ones. If there are particular behaviors that your child struggles with even more than others, and those behaviors are negative, you may feel inclined to gloss over those behaviors. You may do this in an effort to protect your child, to make sure no one looks at him in an unflattering light. But if you gloss over things, the education plan created will not be nearly as useful as if you just buckle down and be honest.

When creating a behavior plan, it is important for your child to be a part of the planning. ADHD children need structure in their lives in and out of school. Your child needs to know exactly what is expected of him in the classroom. Be specific about your expectations. Find out what your child's education goals are, as well as his teacher's goals for him, and combine them with your own goals. Making him a part of the planning process will help to give him a sense of control over his own life. You do not want him to feel as if everyone else is in charge of his life, and he is only a puppet in the play. Bring him into discussions that are suitable for him to hear. For instance, he does not need to be there when you first break the news about his ADHD. There are going to be a lot of questions about his behavior, especially the negative ones, and you do not want your child's self-esteem to take another hit. Instead, bring him with you for the brainstorming meetings to help devise an education plan with expectations he can handle.

Always keep the lines of communication open between you, your child, and his teacher and involved faculty. Contact information needs to be exchanged, including phone numbers, email addresses, and physical addresses. Encourage frequent contact, even if it is simply touching base with a text message. You do not want to consume all of the teacher's time and energy because she has other students to monitor. Come up with specific dates for face-t0-face meetings to discuss your ADHD child's progress. These meetings do not necessarily need to happen once a week. Even a meeting once a month gives you and his teacher the chance to discuss important topics without taking too much of the teacher's time away from her responsibilities.

Take notes of the meetings and keep them with your ADHD child's records at home. Keep track of all communication and what each communication discusses, even simple daily notes home from school that talk about the day's highs and lows. The notes can be useful for discussion with your child's doctor and/or therapist. The notes can also be useful in tracking and monitoring your child's behavior on your own. Reading through the notes will help you see if there is a noticeable improvement over time and areas where the plan may need adjustments. When it comes to dealing with ADHD and behavior plans, you can never have too many observation notes.

WHAT THE TEACHER CAN DO FOR YOUR CHILD

Your ADHD child's teacher plays an important role in his educational success. The teacher spends about 8 hours a day, five days a week with your child throughout the school year. That means she is a vital part of his day-to-day life and a vital member of his education team. Having an ADHD student in her classroom may require certain accommodations geared toward helping the student get through each day. Other students may feel that some of these accommodations or just the way the teacher treats your ADHD child constitute some sort of favoritism. However, there are many different things his teacher can do to accommodate his disorder without making other students feel as if she is showing favoritism.

One essential course of action is to help you determine if your ADHD child needs an Individual Education Program or IEP. An IEP is a specialized service provided to children with qualifying conditions. The IEP is exactly what it says—an individualized plan of education, designed solely for your ADHD child. Rather than your ADHD child having to adhere to the same lesson plan for the rest of the class, instead, he will receive a lesson plan based on his strengths, weaknesses, and educational needs. The IEP is developed by the teachers and parents of the child. Your child's teacher can assist you in finding out if he meets the qualifications for this individual, targeted learning plan. She can also help you through the process of applying for an IEP and getting it approved.

Regardless of whether your child qualifies for an IEP, he is still going to need an educational plan for his time in the classroom. In developing a learning and/or behavior plan for your ADHD child, the teacher needs to be clear about her expectations. However, she must avoid setting the bar too high for your child to reach. No one wants your child to feel as if each day, he is failing. ADHD children often struggle with self-esteem issues. Small, clear goals are a good idea to help your child succeed at a rate with which he can keep up.

Your child's teacher should value communication as much as you do. Giving her all of your contact information, such as a phone number for texting, will ensure that your ADHD child's teacher can always reach you. Perhaps she can even designate a folder specifically for daily notes home. This will provide you with consistent updates on his behaviors and learning skills, along with letting you know when he attains different learning goals. It also gives you the chance to jot down a quick note or question in return for the teacher. Daily note exchanges are ideal for the simple stuff, save the important concerns for phone calls and meetings.

BEHAVIOR AND LEARNING PLAN IDEAS FOR THE TEACHER

We will now discuss a variety of options you and your ADHD child's teacher can include in his education plan. The plan should focus on small goals throughout the school year to avoid overwhelming your child. You both want the goals to be reasonable expectations that keep your child's disorder and educational needs in mind. Ultimate goals – the big ones – should be labeled and discussed while reminding your ADHD child that these are long-term goals—goals that he will work towards over an extended period of time. The plan needs to discuss behaviors, the teacher's expectations within reason, and how behaviors will be reasonably accommodated.

- ADHD children respond well to very specific tasks and goals. Positive reinforcement is the ideal motivator for your ADHD child. The teacher may want to include small rewards for various accomplishments. Even the simplest reward, such as a shiny sticker for good behavior, will motivate your child to succeed. Praising your child for reaching goals and good behaviors will boost his self-esteem and confidence in the classroom. Your child's teacher does not have to exclude other students from this type of positive reinforcement. She can include the entire class in on working towards small, daily rewards. This method keeps the rest of the class from feeling as if your child is getting special treatment. It also prevents your child from possibly feeling singled out because of his disorder.

- In the classroom, your child's teacher can help diminish distractions and lack of focus by making minor adjustments. Placing your ADHD child's desk away from the window helps stop him from always looking outside. Seating him near the teacher's desk is even better. Then, she will be right there to give gentle reminders and instructions. Your child's teacher must pay attention to the students sitting near your child, too. If they seem to distract your child or if he is distracting them, she may have to adjust everyone's seating. Lessons can be given in smaller chunks, rather than all at once to avoid boredom. Your child's teacher can even add movement to some of the lessons, so he is not always stuck in his seat.

- Your ADHD child's habit of interrupting and disrupting can be handled without harsh words or criticism. His teacher might want to create a code word or a hand signal that only your child knows. When he hears this code word or sees the signal, he is reminded to stop and think about his current behavior and it is done without embarrassing him in front of his peers. The word or signal need not be complicated. It just needs to be easy for your child to remember so that when the code is given, he knows how to respond.

- The impulsive nature of your ADHD child requires a detailed schedule and visible behavior plan. He needs the stability of knowing what is going to happen at all times of the school day. Unexpected changes in the daily plan can lead to frustration and outbursts. Your child's teacher needs to write a detailed daily behavior plan that explains rewards and consequences. Keep it clear and simple to ensure that your child understands. Keep the written plan in his line of vision at all times. A quick glance will tell him where he is at in the day's schedule, as well as reminding him of expected behaviors. Consistent, tangible reminders like this written plan help to seal rules and expectations into the mind of your ADHD child.

- When dealing with negative behaviors, his teacher must stick to the written plan and the consequences. Consequences need to be given right away, otherwise, your child may easily forget the associated behavior and not understand why he is getting consequences. His teacher must explain what is happening at that exact moment and why it is happening. If an outburst arises, the teacher needs to remove your ADHD child from the classroom immediately. Taking him out of the stressful situation and into a quiet space, such as the hallway or an empty office, gives him the chance to calm down. Then, the two of them can discuss the situation and the predetermined consequences.

- Younger children with ADHD need more breaks during the school day. They need a chance to move around and play. Your child's teacher can schedule in extra breaks, even if it is only five minutes. This breaks the monotony of the lesson. Recess is also a great time for your ADHD child to burn off some of his extra energy. His teacher should encourage him to participate in games and physical activities during recess. Extra breaks are beneficial for all younger children during the school day. This is another example of accommodations that can be given to all students instead of just your ADHD child.

- Your child's teacher should keep directions and instructions short and sweet. If she gives your ADHD child a list with 10 steps of instructions, it will only take a few minutes for him to be overwhelmed and frustrated. Instead, she can break the directions up into smaller lists. This may mean that she makes one list for him and one list for the rest of the class. This is a small sacrifice to make if it means the day runs smoothly without disruption or outbursts. Again, these small accommodations can be helpful to the rest of the class, so why not share them with all students?

- Your child's teacher must be consistent at all times. She must make it clear to him that she is in charge—she is the authority figure of the classroom. The teacher cannot be soft when it comes to doling out consequences. Otherwise, like any average kid, your child will remember this moment of weakness in the future. From daily schedules to behavior expectations, the teacher has to stay unswerving. The structure will work wonders with your ADHD child and the rest of the class.

ADHD teens often need some accommodations at school, as well. While they do not require shiny stickers on their work, positive words and encouragement can go a long way. As your child grows into a teen, his workload at school is going to change. Reports, term papers, final exams—all of these tasks can be quite intimidating for your ADHD teen. However, there is no reason why his high school teachers cannot make a few minor changes with him in mind. Just as with your younger child's teacher, you need to get all of his high school teachers on the team and on the same page.

Just as younger children respond better to smaller tasks and assignments, so do teenage children. Your ADHD teens teachers can provide him with assignments and instructions that are broken into smaller, more manageable pieces. Each set of instructions is a minor goal for your teen to reach. Just because he is older now does not mean he no longer needs verbal recognition of his accomplishments, even the minor ones. His teachers should give him praise when he hits a small goal to encourage him not to give up. Even if the assignment is a ten-page term paper, single-spaced, and including a bibliography, your ADHD teen is still capable of completing it with success. Once the assignment is broken down into smaller goals, your teen will see that each goal is attainable and will lead him to the ultimate goal—the successful completion of the entire term paper.

ADHD teens in high school may not be familiar with certain learning skills that will help them in each class. Your teen's teachers may want to meet with him after school to give him additional help and instruction. This is also a good time for them to work with your teen on helpful skills, such as how to take notes during a lecture and how to study for an exam. These skills may come easy to the average high school teen, but your ADHD teen already struggles with organization and staying focused. Being taught specific methods of note-taking and studying in a way that is easy for him to understand will help your ADHD teen achieve his academic goals. Being taught these skills before or after school ensures that he is not embarrassed in front of his peers by his need for extra help.

Hyperactive ADHD teens with lots of energy could flourish in a team sport. His teachers can discuss the various extracurricular activities with your teen to help him decide if he wants to participate. Not only will it help him learn more socialization skills, but he will also discover what it is like to be a part of a group. The group, which is the team, is working together to achieve one common goal. Whether it be a touchdown or a home run, your ADHD teen will have the chance to help his team reach their goal. Sports like basketball, football, soccer, and even wrestling will give your teen a chance to release energy and exercise in a fun, competitive environment. If your ADHD teen worries about not being good enough for a team, discuss his options with the different coaches to discover where he fits in the best.

For ADHD teens, disciplinary actions and consequences differ from those of younger children. High school can be a tough environment to withstand, even for the strongest teen. Your teen's teachers need to keep the ADHD in mind when dealing with negative behaviors. This does not mean that your teen requires special treatment, or that he will be allowed to get away with breaking the rules. It simply means that the punishments need to fit the crimes so that your ADHD teen has a clear understanding of why he is receiving a certain consequence. Discipline, even in the school setting, is not always one-size-fits-all. Every child and teen are unique, and some situations call for a different approach.

PARENTAL TIPS FOR EDUCATIONAL SUCCESS AT HOME

Now you know what you need to do as far as addressing your child's ADHD with his school, encouraging and participating in open lines of communication, and how you can participate in creating a learning plan. These are all essential actions to take for your child's educational success. However, that is not all you can do. There are lots of things you can do at home to assist your child in managing his ADHD in conjunction with the school. Providing accommodations at home keeps the educational process in both places consistent. It will not do your ADHD child any good to have a structured environment at school and pure chaos at home.

- One of the greatest gifts you can give to your ADHD child is a love for reading. Studies have repeatedly demonstrated the importance of reading. To help prevent your child from struggling with reading and comprehension, take charge at home from a young age. Read together every day at a specific time. Make story time fun and entertaining. Create character voices to keep your ADHD child intrigued. Ask him questions throughout the book, such as asking what he thinks will happen next. Younger ADHD children will get a kick out of helping you physically act out the storyline— an added bonus is your ADHD child burns some additional energy.

- Help your ADHD child succeed with homework, not by completing it for him, but by teaching the skills he needs to do it on his own. When he has questions or appears to be struggling, you can walk him through the steps one at a time, showing him the way to arrive at the solution on his own. When your child comes home with a messy backpack full of papers in disarray, it is time to organize. File folders are a handy tool for teaching organizational skills to your ADHD child. Label each file clearly so that he always knows where to find particular papers.

- Talk to his teacher about giving him one folder that is solely for homework assignments. This visual aid tells him with only a glance if he has homework. An empty homework folder means an evening free for other activities. It will also keep you informed on homework stats. His teacher simply needs to put homework papers in the homework folder each day.

- Create a homework schedule and checklist. Visual reminders are vital tools for children with ADHD. A checklist of homework tasks that your child can review every evening can help him stay on top of his studies. Your ADHD child also needs a specific place just for homework—somewhere quiet where he can work without distractions. The schedule should include specific times for homework sessions, as well as breaks. For example, a schedule might go as follows:

- 3:30 pm – Arrive home, place the daily folder on the table, check the homework folder for assignments, and place the homework folder on the desk

- 3:40 pm – Snack time

- 4:00 pm – Meet me at your desk to organize the day's homework

- 4:10 pm – Begin your homework one paper at a time – REMEMBER: I'm here to answer your questions and help when needed

- 4:30 pm – Take a break, stretch your legs, get a quick drink

- 4:40 pm – Continue homework assignments

- 5:00 pm – Take another break

- 5:10 pm – Back to work OR if homework is completed, we will review it together

As you can see, that simple schedule specifies every aspect of your ADHD child's after school routine. It can easily be adjusted if his homework takes longer than an hour. On days when your child has no homework, you can create another schedule with a non-homework routine. This kind of structure ensures that your child always knows what he should be doing at any given time of the evening. If he forgets or gets distracted, just remind him to check the schedule. Any schedule you create can be as simple or detailed as you want. Include your ADHD child in on the planning. That way, he knows that his needs and wants are heard, and he will be less likely to complain about the schedule later.

Even though ADHD is going to impact your child's education, the power lies with you, your child, and his teacher to make it a positive impact. Working together as a team and confronting ADHD head-on is the best way to guide your child through his school years, reaching goals and achievements along the way. Planning, schedules, routines, structure, and some accommodating will ensure that your ADHD child's school days are filled with learning, activities, socialization, and the satisfaction of a job well done.

CHAPTER 4:

WHEN AND HOW TO SEEK A PROFESSIONAL DIAGNOSIS OF ADHD

At this point in the book, you have learned a great deal about ADHD. You now know exactly what ADHD is, potential causes, possible symptoms and associated conditions, how ADHD can affect your family, and how it impacts school. While this is all a lot of information to absorb, understanding every aspect of ADHD is only going to help you to help your child. One of three things led you to this book.

1. You already have an ADHD child.

2. You suspect your child may have ADHD.

3. You are a proactive parent learning about a very common condition "just in case."

If you already know that your child has ADHD, you are here to learn as much as you can about it so you can assist your child. If you think you might have an ADHD child, you are here to learn about the disorder so you can decide if you should worry. Finally, you may have no pressing concerns about ADHD in your child, you just know it is common, and you want to be educated and aware. No matter which reason brings you here, it is time to discuss when and how you should pursue a medical diagnosis of ADHD in your child.

DOES MY CHILD HAVE ADHD?

In today's world, it seems as if there are more disorders of the brain than there ever were in the past. This explosion of conditions and disorders and special needs only adds to the worries every parent has for their children. While there is no need to get yourself in a frenzy worrying about every possible condition, it is okay to be aware, be observant, and be informed. This is especially true when it comes to ADHD because it is one of the most common disorders affecting children today.

In that case, does your child have ADHD? Should you be worried about ADHD? When and how should you watch for symptoms? When is it time for a professional evaluation? How do you even get a medical professional to evaluate your child for ADHD? These are just a few of the questions that many parents have. Asking these questions and educating yourself on the answers will ensure that you—as a parent—are informed and prepared in case ADHD knocks on the door.

WHEN AND HOW TO WATCH FOR ADHD SYMPTOMS

Earlier, you learned about classic and most common symptoms of ADHD in general. You then learned in-depth information about ADHD symptoms, as well as possible conditions associated with the disorder. You learned what symptoms to look for in both different age groups and grade levels of children. The symptoms and associated conditions were discussed in detail as well. The next step in understanding ADHD is learning when and how you should monitor your child for symptoms.

Knowing when you should begin watching for symptoms of ADHD can be hard to pinpoint. First, every child is different. While studies indicate that the predisposition to develop ADHD is within your child from birth, this does not mean he will definitely develop the disorder, or that the symptoms will manifest at a specific age. Not knowing when to watch for symptoms is worrisome. Should you be observant when your child is a baby? Should you start monitoring his behavior when he is a toddler? Perhaps you should not worry at all until he starts school. It can all be quite confusing for any parent. The following tips will help you decide when is the best time to watch for ADHD symptoms in your child.

- **Infants and babies** – Having an infant or a baby under the age of 2 diagnosed with ADHD is highly unlikely. At this age, there simply is not a feasible method of watching for symptoms. There are not even realistic symptoms to watch for at these very young ages. The best thing you can do during the first 24 months of your child's life is to simply be a parent and nurture and love your baby. There are no classic symptoms to observe. Babies' reactions are very instinctual during this time—primal, even. There is no method to the madness. If there is a family history of ADHD, you can prepare yourself for things to watch for when your child is older.

- **Toddlers** – When your child reaches the age of 2, he is now considered a toddler. He has more control over his actions—although, not very much—and he is a sponge for knowledge. ADHD symptoms can begin to develop in children as young as 2–4 years old. The problem with observing for symptoms during the toddler years is all toddlers tend to exhibit the classic signs of ADHD: being hyperactive, lacking impulse control, and being inattentive. Toddlers are naturally self-centered and have a very short attention span. Have you ever noticed that when a toddler wants something, he wants it now and has no patience for waiting? Have you experienced those "terrible twos?" Determining whether your toddler's behaviors are normal or a cause for concern is difficult. The best thing you can watch for during these early years are telltale signs of the 3 classic ADHD symptoms.

    o *Hyperactivity*: Toddlers are active, but if your toddler is overly active, it could be a symptom. For example, he may fidget, wiggle, squirm and fuss each and every time he has to sit down. If you notice that he cannot sit still at mealtime or when you are holding him and reading a book, make a note, especially if this behavior happens every day. It may seem as if your child has a motor that will not stop, keeping him in motion all day to the point of exhaustion.

- o **Impulsivity**: Yes, toddlers are impulsive, little people. However, if you feel like your child takes his impulsivity to an extreme, it may be time to consider ADHD. Some signs could be throwing multiple emotional tantrums several times a day. His natural impatience from his age could seem as if it is on steroids. In other words, he has absolutely no patience and tolerance for sharing, taking turns, or even just being around other toddlers.

- o **Inattention**: The level of attentiveness is probably the most difficult ADHD symptom to determine during toddlerhood. Toddlers normally struggle with sticking with any single activity for an extended period of time. Toddlers are also easily distracted and often do not listen. However, you can watch for telltale signs, such as if your 3-year-old seems to have trouble following simple instructions. For example, at 3 years, your toddler should be able to take an item to the garbage or put a toy in the toy box. If it appears that he is not understanding simple commands, there may be an underlying reason, including ADHD.

Again, an ADHD diagnosis is very difficult during the toddler years. Take note of any behaviors that you feel go beyond normal. Keep an eye out for physical delays, such as struggling to hop on one foot by the time he is 4 years old. Also, toddlers normally have some sort of separation anxiety that includes a healthy fear of strangers. If your little one does not seem to have any stranger-danger fears, it may be a warning sign of ADHD. Observe your toddler with others his own age, and see how his behaviors compare to their behaviors. If you have major concerns after careful observation over a length of time, take those concerns to his pediatrician.

- **Older children and teens (5 and up)** – Watching for ADHD symptoms in children over the age of 5 is actually much easier than trying to make a determination any younger. The average age when a child is most often diagnosed with ADHD is 7 years old. Even though warning signs may manifest at a younger age, it is easier to pinpoint the disorder when the child is older. One reason it is easier to become aware of a possible disorder is because your child is now in school. Behaviors at home and at school can often vary. While you might fear he has ADHD because he is a terror at home, he might just be an absolute angel at school. However, if he exhibits hyperactivity, inattentiveness, and lack of impulse control at home and at school, it could definitely be ADHD.

ADHD is not on a time schedule. It is not going to automatically appear at any certain age. Your child may display signs when he is 6 or 7 years of age, or the symptoms may appear when he is 12. That is why you have to be aware and observant, especially if there is a potential genetic link. You and your child's teacher, regardless of his age, can join forces and track his behaviors. Enlisting in the aid of his teacher will provide you with information about his behavior when you are not present. It is as easy as taking notes of certain behaviors at home and in the classroom. Then, you and his teacher can compare notes to determine if there might be a need for ADHD evaluation.

Now that you know more about observing and tracking your child's possible symptoms at every age group, it is time to discuss the next step. If you feel that there is a cause for ADHD concerns at any age, prepare to have your child evaluated by a medical professional. Do not attempt any medicinal forms of ADHD treatments at home. This includes both prescription drugs and homeopathic supplements. Giving your child someone else's ADHD medication is dangerous and illegal. Supplements are not regulated by the FDA, and they should not be administered without a doctor's approval. Attempting to treat ADHD without a medical diagnosis could put your child's health at risk, especially if he does not have ADHD at all.

GETTING A PROFESSIONAL DIAGNOSIS

So, you are now at the point where you feel that your child may have ADHD. The first step in this determination is to seek medical advice. Start by gathering all of your written concerns and any concerns or recommendations from his teacher if he is currently in school. You want to have good records of observed behaviors over an extended period of time—at least six months. It is also important to have his teacher's observations because a medical diagnosis of ADHD is normally not given unless the behaviors are observed in two completely different settings, such as at home and at school. Medical professionals use these different environmental observations to help them determine if your child is unable to control his behavior anywhere. There are some cases in which a child simply acts out at home.

Now that you have your records and his teacher's records, it is time to make that first phone call. Keep in mind that ADHD is not something that can be diagnosed with a throat swab or a blood test. It involves a full evaluation and observation of your child and his behaviors. Contact your child's primary physician. It does not matter if his doctor is a pediatrician or a general practitioner. Make certain that you stipulate that the appointment is to discuss the possibility of ADHD. This gives your child's doctor a chance to prepare for the discussion. At the appointment, present your written records from home and from school. Voice all of your concerns with your child's doctor. Include any family history of ADHD because genetics can, of course, increase your child's risk of developing the disorder.

At this point, your child's doctor is likely to take one of two routes in evaluating your child for ADHD. First, the doctor may have paperwork for you to fill out. This paperwork will include questionnaires about your child's behaviors. There is usually a long list of questions to answer. The questions will ask about specific behaviors and symptoms and how often they are observed in your child. For instance, the question may inquire about difficulty going to sleep and difficulty staying asleep. These are both two separate symptoms. Your answer choices are typically in the form of some type of scale. An example would be all the time, frequently, occasionally, and never. The doctor will provide a specific questionnaire for you, as well as one designed for your child's teacher. As mentioned earlier, the behaviors need to be observed in two different settings to make an ADHD diagnosis.

You will need to come back at a later date to return the questionnaires. The answers you and your child's teacher give will help the doctor determine if an ADHD diagnosis is warranted. Should the doctor make this decision, he will discuss treatment options with you and your child. Bear in mind that this is a rather expedited form of diagnosis. While it is perfectly valid, it does not include an in-depth, personal observation of your child. However, the questionnaires are quite specific and designed to determine the existence of ADHD. It is imperative that the answers are honest.

If your child's doctor takes the second route, he will want to refer your child to a specialist who will evaluate your child for ADHD. You can expect a referral to a child psychologist or psychiatrist. It may seem overwhelming to think about having your child evaluated by a mental health professional. Do not panic if this is the doctor's plan of action. This does not mean that your child is "crazy" and destined for a life of mental health problems. The days of feeling shame or embarrassment at the idea of visiting a "shrink" are gone. It is now 2019, and society understands the importance of good mental health in addition to good physical health.

Child psychologists and psychiatrists specialize in various disorders, including ADHD. Both professionals are able to medically diagnose ADHD. One primary difference between psychologists and psychiatrists is that psychologists are unable to prescribe prescription medications. However, if a psychologist gives the diagnosis of ADHD in your child, he can then refer you to a psychiatrist for medications if that is part of the treatment plan. You can also just take the diagnosis back to your child's primary physician who is also able to prescribe medications.

The plan of action for an ADHD evaluation with a psychologist or psychiatrist can vary. A typical scenario involves an initial appointment for you, the parent. This is when you will start all of the paperwork and there is a lot of paperwork. You will have to provide basic information, such as birthdate, insurance, allergies to medicines, emergency contact, family history, etc. These forms are necessary for all new patients. You can also expect various forms of questionnaires for you and for your child's teacher. The specialist will discuss your concerns with you during the appointment. You will then arrange for a second appointment to return the paperwork. This second appointment is normally when the specialist will meet your child.

At the second appointment, return all of the questionnaires you and the teacher answered. This is a good time to turn over your written records that led to your concerns. Bring your child with you. The specialist will meet with both of you at the same time for a discussion about ADHD and what you and your child can expect from the evaluation. The evaluation normally consists of more than just answering questions on forms. The specialist will need to spend time with your child alone so that he can interact with your child and make his own observations. This separate meeting may or may not occur at the second appointment. However, you should expect future appointments to proceed in this manner: a meeting and discussion with you, your child, and the specialist together, followed by an allotted amount of time for the specialist to talk to and observe your child alone. The entire evaluation process to determine if ADHD is present should not take more than a few appointments.

Once it is determined that your child does have ADHD, the specialist will give you an official diagnosis. At this point, he may suggest continued appointments for therapy and counseling that will benefit both you and your child. These additional appointments would be part of the ADHD treatment plan. These therapeutic sessions allow the specialist to continue monitoring your child and his progress with managing ADHD. The sessions will also give you the opportunity to discuss additional concerns or questions you might have during the initial treatment plan. Counseling sessions are a part of behavior management, which is extremely beneficial in the treatment of ADHD. The specialist will teach you how to manage behaviors at home, and he will teach your child how to self-manage his own behavior through various methods. Whether or not you choose to continue these therapy sessions depends on how you have decided to treat your child's ADHD.

After being professionally diagnosed with ADHD, your child needs treatment. Leaving ADHD untreated is practically child abuse. When you know that your child has a condition, it is your responsibility to seek medical treatment, mental health treatment, or even both. If your child was sick with a fever and severe sore throat that turned out to be strep throat, would you just disregard the diagnosis and expect it to heal itself? Of course not! You would follow the doctor's orders and obtain the necessary antibiotics to treat the illness. The same train of thought applies to ADHD. Your child has been medically diagnosed with ADHD, and he exhibits numerous symptoms of the disorder. Are you going to ignore the advice of medical professionals and decline treatment? While ADHD is not an illness like strep throat that can be cured with antibiotics, it is a condition that can be treated in a variety of ways. It is your duty as your child's caregiver and protector to do whatever it takes to provide treatment for him.

A treatment plan can be determined in conjunction with the specialist and/or your child's primary physician. While an actual diagnosis is likely to be a bit frightening for you and your child, the important thing to keep in mind is that you now have an explanation for all of his behaviors—and it is not your fault. It is okay for you, as the parent, to actually feel some sort of relief because you finally have a valid answer. Even though ADHD is not something you would wish on your child, knowing that he has the disorder allows both of you to take the next step, which is to figure out the best methods of treating the ADHD. With medical discoveries and treatment methods consistently improving every year, it is only a matter of time before your child will start to feel better about himself, behave better at home and at school, and have a better quality of life.

CHAPTER 5:

TREATING ADHD

When your child is diagnosed with ADHD, designing a treatment plan is the first course of action. You will quickly discover that there are numerous methods for treating ADHD. The goal of the treatment plan should be to lessen and manage the symptoms of ADHD. Up to this point, your child has been living with ADHD on his own. Untreated ADHD can cause a child to feel a wide range of emotions that are more intense than the average child. He has likely felt immense frustration and confusion. He has likely battled with feeling completely out of control. The restlessness and extra energy have disrupted his mind and his body. There are probably times when he felt judged by others due to his behaviors, even made to feel like he was just a "bad kid." Even though ADHD does not have a cure, with the right treatment plan, your child will no longer have to struggle and suffer.

ADHD TREATMENT OPTIONS

Deciding how to treat your child's ADHD can be a daunting task. There is a myriad of options available. Prescription medications have been shown to be one of the most effective treatments. Approximately 80% of children and adults with ADHD respond to prescription medication. Taking a closer look at proven, available medications can help you decide where to begin. No matter which medication you ultimately choose, expect a period of trial-and-error. People respond differently to medications; the pill that works for one child may not work for your ADHD child. It can take several months of trying different medications before you find the one that works. The looming questions remain: Which ADHD medication is best for my child?

Prescription Treatment

There is a multitude of prescription medications available for ADHD. The medications increase the amounts of certain neurotransmitters in the brain: norepinephrine and/or dopamine. These medications fall into three categories as follows:

- **Stimulant drugs** – Stimulants have a proven track record of over 50 years of success in the treatment of ADHD. These types of drugs increase both norepinephrine and dopamine. These neurotransmitters help an ADHD child to focus and concentrate better. One of the benefits of stimulants is that they work quickly. The effect is going to be noticeable almost immediately. Stimulant medications can be designed to release all at once, or they can be designed to release over an extended amount of time. The effective time period of stimulants can range from as little as 4 hours or as much as 12 hours.

- Immediate-release medications that last from 4–6 hours may aid your child in getting through the school day. While he may need an additional dose during school, you can give the faculty permission to administer the dose as prescribed. Extended-release stimulants can be just as effective through the school day, and their effects can carry over into the evening. These types of stimulants are good for children that more than a boost to get through the school day.

- Common ADHD stimulant drugs include Ritalin, Adderall, Vyvanse, Concerta, Daytrana, and Focalin. You have probably heard of some of these medications. Ritalin has long been prescribed for ADHD, and it has been proven successful in many children. Years of medical research on the effect of ADHD in the brain has provided many other stimulant options besides Ritalin. Stimulants are usually a doctor's first line of defense in treating ADHD with medication.

- **Non-stimulant drugs** – Non-stimulant drugs are just that—not stimulating. These types of drugs increase norepinephrine in your child's brain. Non-stimulants have been shown to help a child's memory and attention span. These medications do not work as quickly as stimulant drugs, but their effects can last for as long as 24 hours. The long-lasting effects of non-stimulants may be an advantage to you and your child because you will not have to worry about multiple doses in a day or the medication wearing off at the wrong time.

- Common ADHD non-stimulant drugs include Intuniv, Strattera, Pamelor, and Kapvay. Your child's doctor may prescribe a non-stimulant medication if stimulant drugs have not helped your child's symptoms or if the side-effects of stimulants have proven too much for your child. The doctor may also decide to use both stimulants and non-stimulants to treat ADHD symptoms.

- **Antidepressant drugs** – Although not as commonly used as stimulants and non-stimulants, antidepressants such as Wellbutrin, Norpramin, Tofranil, and Aventyl are sometimes helpful in the treatment of ADHD. Although the FDA does not specifically recommend antidepressants for ADHD, some doctors have found that when used in conjunction with stimulants, antidepressants help manage the disorder.

While prescription medications may sound like the quick and easy answer to the problem, it is imperative that you weigh the advantages and disadvantages of using these drugs. You already know the most beneficial advantages—reducing and managing the symptoms with a pill. Even though it can take months of observing your child on different medications before finding the one that really works, the time will be well-spent, right? Because once you find the best medication, your problems are over! Unfortunately, that is not always the case.

Just as with any medication on the market, prescription ADHD medications come with the risk of various side effects. These side effects can be mild, moderate, or severe. Every child responds differently to medications, so discovering how your child is going to respond requires putting him on the medication and watching for side effects. This can actually be quite a nerve-wracking experience for you as a parent because you do not know what to expect. It can also be a difficult and even traumatic experience for your child if the side effects prove to be quite severe.

Common side effects of stimulant and non-stimulant medications may include the following:

- stomachaches
- headaches
- dry mouth
- decreased appetite resulting in weight loss
- trouble sleeping
- irritability
- nervousness

While these potential side effects may seem like a minor risk, there are more severe side effects that could occur. These severe side effects may include the following:

- allergic reactions
- high blood pressure
- visual and audible hallucinations
- increased risk of heart problems

- seizures

- suicidal thoughts and/or actions

In fact, Strattera actually has a black-box warning because studies have indicated that children and teenagers taking Strattera are more likely to have suicidal thoughts. Antidepressants have also been shown to increase the risk of suicide in children and teens. Although these severe side effects are rare and do not occur in every child, you have to ask yourself one question. Are you willing to take the chance, no matter how small, that your child may have a severe side effect? If you decide that medication is an option, be ready for the sometimes daunting task of watching for side effects. Each prescription medication has its own list of advantages and disadvantages. Take the time to research each medication thoroughly before making your decision.

It cannot be said enough times—treatment is trial-and-error. Your child needs the right medication at the optimal dosage and schedule, as well as with the fewest side effects. You could observe the desired results in the first month on the first choice of medication. It could also take six months and six different medications before you see results. There is even the possibility that medications will not help your child at all. Discuss the options in-depth with your child's doctor and do your own research. Do not hesitate to voice any concerns and questions about each possible option before and during each trial stage. Communication between you and your child's doctor is extremely important during the first stages of prescription treatments.

Prescription Alternatives
While it is easy to assume that prescriptions are the most likely to help your ADHD child, it is important to consider other methods of treatment that do not include prescriptions. Many parents are quite leery of giving drugs to their child, especially a young child. Even though the drug is recommended and prescribed by a medical professional, parents can be fearful of "doping" their

child or of the dreaded "zombie" effect. You do not want to change the overall personality of your child. You simply want to help him manage the overwhelming symptoms of ADHD. The thought of putting prescription drugs into your child's system can be frightening. There are so many possible side effects, and there is no guarantee that any of the medications will work for your child. Many parents have turned to a treatment plan that does not include prescription medications.

Alternative methods of treating ADHD often include diet and lifestyle changes, increased physical activity and exercise, and meditation. Even a method of "brain-training" that teaches the brain to be more focused and less impulsive can be utilized in place of medications. Learning more about alternative approaches can aid you in designing the right ADHD treatment plan for your child. You may decide to utilize alternative methods in conjunction with other methods of treatment.

- **Dietary changes** – Changing your child's diet to increase his intake of specific nutrients, complex carbohydrates, and proteins can help his brain perform at its best and help control his mood swings.

    - Omega-3 fatty acids found in fish, such as sardines and salmon, feed the brain's fat.

    - Foods rich in magnesium, such as avocado, soy, leafy greens, and dark chocolate, can aid in improving mood swings, concentration, and sleep patterns.

    - Increasing protein in your child's diet can help boost attention and decrease hyperactivity.

    - Foods like whole grains, legumes, and vegetables, which are high in fiber, can help even out your child's energy levels.

- Supplements that include fish oil, magnesium, vitamin C, vitamin B6, zinc, and iron may be beneficial because these vitamins and minerals aid in the production and regulation of the brain's neurotransmitters. Supplements also make it easier for your child to gain the benefits of the minerals and vitamins without having to eat foods that he may not enjoy. Ensure that your child's doctor approves the supplements before you try them.

Limiting and avoiding certain foods can also aid in treating the behaviors of ADHD. You do not have to go overboard and cut out the majority of your child's diet. You do not want to overwhelm your ADHD child with extreme changes in his diet all at once. A few, minor changes can make a difference.

- Keep your child's sugar intake to a minimum.

- Try to avoid specific food preservatives and food colorings, including D&C Yellow No. 10, sodium benzoate, and FD&C Red No. 40, Yellow No. 5, and Yellow No. 6.

- Steer clear of foods that may be a possible allergen, such as chocolate, eggs, and salicylate foods like chili powder and tomatoes.

Dietary changes alone may not manage all of your child's ADHD symptoms but they can be a good place to start. You can also just include dietary changes with other methods of treatment. The best scenario is that the changes to your child's diet help the ADHD symptoms. The worst scenario is that your child simply has a healthier diet. Dietary changes can be a win-win situation for your ADHD child.

- **Exercise and physical activity** – An ADHD diagnosis means that it is time to get your child up and moving. It is a proven fact that exercise increases mood-improving endorphins in the brain. Exercise also increases the brain's dopamine and serotonin levels which aid in attention and focusing. Exercise and physical activity also give your ADHD child an interactive task upon which to concentrate.

  For example, many ADHD children benefit from martial arts, tai-chi, ballet, and yoga. These activities require mental strength and concentration. Your child has to pay attention to learn the yoga poses, martial arts moves, and ballet dances. The calming meditation that comes with yoga and tai-chi have also shown to improve anxiety and hyperactivity. The meditative methods teach your child new methods of calming himself at any time.

- **Green therapy** – This type of therapy is simple. All you need to do is have your child spend time in the lush, green environment of nature. Studies indicate that spending as little as 20 minutes a day in a green environment improves the symptoms of ADHD in adults and children. It not only has a soothing, calming effect on your child, it can also help with improving concentration and attention. A green environment does not mean you have to take a daily trip to a national forest. Consider visiting a local greenhouse, walking a nature trail at the park, or spending some time on the riverbank. There are plenty of environments outside in nature from which to choose.

- **Brain-training** – While this may sound like something out of a science fiction novel, brain-training is a real thing. While science has yet to determine if it truly helps with ADHD symptoms, many parents notice improvements in attention and memory. Brain-training involves the use of specifically-designed software programs. Cogmed is a program that helps improve your child's working memory.

The working memory lets your child remember information short-term so that he can perform a task; for example, remembering an address or phone number. Other brain-training software programs are designed to train the brain to be less impulsive and to pay more attention. Your child will "play" what appear to be video games. These games help him to exercise parts of his brain that may not be performing at their best.

- **EEG biofeedback** – This particular alternative ADHD treatment is a technological method of treatment. Your child will attend an EEG biofeedback session, which is a neurotherapy that measures his brain waves. This means that he will be hooked up to equipment such as a cap that is lined with electrodes. The cap will measure his brain waves as he is asked to perform a specific task. The task may involve playing a video game or solving a problem. The point of the EEG biofeedback session is to teach your child to produce the brain waves that are associated with focusing. Your child will not experience any pain, and the sessions do not last longer than 30 minutes but this is a very expensive form of treatment. Each session can cost several thousand dollars—even as much as $5,000 per session.

These are just a few of the alternative, non-prescription methods utilized to treat ADHD. If you are strongly against giving your child prescription medication, you need to research these and other alternative treatments. Discuss alternative methods with your child's doctor. You may even decide to incorporate the two together—medication and alternative methods—into your child's ADHD treatment plan. Just as with the medications, these alternatives are trial-and-error. Some methods may show positive results, while others do not help with his ADHD symptoms at all. If you choose to go the alternative route, be patient and diligent with your methods. Many of these alternatives are lifestyle changes, which means your life will change in conjunction with your child's life.

One more non-prescription method of treating ADHD is therapy. While prescription medication designed specifically for ADHD is usually an effective treatment, it is important to understand that it is not the only treatment. Therapy programs designed to teach your child how to manage his symptoms are also effective. In fact, the American Academy of Pediatrics recommends a combined treatment plan of medication and therapy for children ages 6 years and older. For children younger than 6 years, therapy alone is usually the preferred method of treatment before prescription medications. In order to truly understand the benefits of therapy in managing ADHD symptoms, it is necessary to take a much closer look at this treatment option.

CHAPTER 6:

THERAPY AND COUNSELING AS AN ADHD TREATMENT

Therapy is a non-prescription method of treating ADHD. Therapy is often included in an ADHD treatment plan to be used in conjunction with medication. If you do not want your child on medication, you can still utilize therapy in conjunction with alternative treatment methods. While medication has been successful, recent studies have indicated that therapy can be just as effective. It has been shown that ADHD children treated with therapy first actually demonstrated faster progress than those that started treatment with medication.

Therapy is beneficial with or without other treatment methods. Therapy does not have to be a visit to the psychiatrist every week. Even weekly counseling sessions at school or with a trained professional have proven to be beneficial in treating ADHD. There are different forms of therapy that you can use for your child. There are even forms of therapy that will benefit the entire family. Therapy focuses on the specific ADHD behaviors and the emotional aspect of ADHD, providing both the child and the family with coping skills.

BEHAVIOR THERAPY

The most common type of therapy utilized in the treatment of ADHD is behavior therapy. To put it simply, behavior therapy changes behaviors through conditioning. The therapist will meet with your child and begin to teach him how to change his behaviors. Behavior therapy focuses on positive reinforcement and consequences. The therapist will help your child to modify his behaviors. Each behavior will be addressed and solutions will be offered. Over time, you will notice your child's behavior changing.

There are different things you can expect in behavior therapy. First, the focus will be on small, specific behaviors. Trying to modify numerous behaviors at once is simply setting your child up for failure. Each session will discuss a specific behavior and how your child can make small changes to modify the behavior. You can also expect a behavior plan. This plan should be simple and to the point. Much like the after-school schedule discussed earlier, the behavior plan needs to be very specific. The therapist will help you determine which behaviors to focus on for the plan. The following tips will help you prepare a successful behavior plan.

- Determine which behaviors you want to focus on with your child. Do not be vague in your choices. For example, if you need your child to go to bed at a specific time each night, make that one goal. Do not make the goal too big for your child to achieve, such as getting up at 7 am and being completely ready for school by 7:45. This is simply too much at once for your ADHD child to remember. Take baby steps to achieve the ultimate goal.

- Be realistic in your expectations from your ADHD child. He has been battling ADHD for a while now. Behavior modification does not happen overnight. It happens through conditioning, which is the repetitive performance of an action until it becomes a habit. If your child has always struggled to go to bed on time, the struggle is not going to change with one try.

- Utilize a chart detailing each behavior for the week that you want your ADHD child to work on. As each behavior is slowly modified until it is changed, the chart can be changed to different behaviors. The visual chart provides your ADHD child with something he can see and focus on every day. Use stickers on his "good" days as a little bit of positive reinforcement. You can even add a checklist he can use to check off each accomplishment through the day.

- Provide positive reinforcement for every accomplished behavior modification. This means that when your child does manage to make it to bed on time, reward him the next day. The rewards can be the positive stickers applied to his behavior chart. Positive reinforcement can even just be in the form of enthusiastic appreciation and praise in addition to the sticker. After he collects so many stickers, then he gets a simple reward, like a trip for ice cream or an inexpensive toy.

- Provide a consequence for forgotten behavior modifications. This means that when your child fails to be in bed on time, a consequence has to be given. Consequences do not have to be mean. It can be as simple as not providing the praise and appreciation you gave as positive reinforcement. It can be removing a privilege. Make sure that the punishment fits the crime. For failing to be in bed on time, the consequence can be given immediately when you see that your ADHD child is still up and running. Firmly remind him that it is past bedtime, and let him know he will not receive a positive sticker on the chart.

- Praise him when he gets it right because if an ADHD child does not feel that his efforts are recognized, he is likely to slip right back into old habits. You do not have to throw a party in celebration each time your child gets something right, verbal acknowledgment of his success is sufficient. Save the celebrations for when he reaches long-term behavior goals.

- Be consistent with the reward and consequence plan. If he achieves his goal, give him his reward. Do not put it off or change it at the last minute. This will only frustrate and disappoint your ADHD child, making him less likely to want to try to modify his behaviors. The same is true for consequences. You have to be consistent. It is very easy for parents of all children to ignore a bad behavior or not follow through with a consequence. You simply have to follow through with consequences, or your ADHD child's behaviors will never change.

- Remember your part in the behavior plan. Do not expect your child to no longer need reminders. Instead, focus on giving him fewer reminders. Using our bedtime example, if you normally have to tell your child more than 10 times to go to bed, make the goal to only remind him 3 times. Then, if after three reminders he still is not in bed, it is time for a consequence.

- Your part also includes being patient. If you are not patient with the modification plan, it is destined to fail. Why? Because your ADHD child will know that you are frustrated with him. ADHD children can be quick to give up if they feel frustrated or defeated. All children pick up on the mood and energies emanating from parents. Be patient and positive with your child.

- As your child succeeds with a behavior modification, you can change the behavior plan and start focusing on a different behavior. If your ADHD child shows signs of reverting back to an old behavior, you should only have to give gentle reminders to keep him on track.

The behavior therapist will continue to have sessions with your child to monitor his progress. The chart makes it easy to track his behavior for a week. Then, you can just show the chart to the therapist at each visit. If progress is not being made, the therapist will help you adjust the behavior plan and goals. The behavior modification is not just for your child; it is also applicable to you. The therapist will educate you on how to enforce the behavior plan at home. She will teach you how to set small goals for your ADHD child and how to help him achieve them. If you have spent the past few years having a short temper with your child because of his behaviors, she will teach you how to modify your own reactions.

The total behavior modification process will last as long as you want it to last. Once you have a firm grasp on your ADHD child's behavior plan, how to make it, and how to enforce it, your sessions with the therapist will decrease. As your child makes progress, he may only need to be seen two times a month. Ideally, your child will eventually no longer need therapy sessions— because you and your child will have learned how to modify his behaviors on your own. When your child no longer has to have sessions with the behavior therapist, you will know that he is on the right path to overcoming his behaviors with long-term results.

OTHER TYPES OF THERAPY

There are many different types of therapy that can help your ADHD child and the family unit manage the behaviors that come with the disorder. While behavior therapy is the most commonly used ADHD therapy, there are other options for you to consider. There are also different therapeutic options for you, the parent, and for the family. Different types of therapy give you choices in your method of managing your child's behavior. Therapy, just like medication, is not a one-size-fits-all form of treatment. Your child may benefit from one type of therapy more than another, or he may even require two or three types of therapy to achieve the best results.

COGNITIVE BEHAVIORAL THERAPY

This type of therapy is focused more on the thoughts and feelings of your ADHD child. It is probably more like the type of therapy you imagine in your head—a talking session with the therapist. It is a time for talking about behaviors, how your ADHD child feels, and how to help him cope with his feelings. Cognitive therapy is designed to change the way your child thinks about himself. It will turn his negative thoughts and feelings into positive thoughts and feelings. For every negative feeling he has, the therapist will help him to look at it in a positive light.

One example could be if your child feels discouraged at school because he often forgets to turn in his work, resulting in poor grades. The focus of the cognitive therapy session would be on the behavior: forgetfulness. The therapist will discuss the reasons behind his forgetfulness. For instance, is he being distracted by someone or something in the classroom on a regular basis? Then, she will help your ADHD child to figure out a way to deal with the behavior. This could be having him ask his teacher to move his seat so he will no longer be distracted. When the strategies to change a behavior do not work, the therapist and your child will find new strategies to try.

Cognitive behavioral therapy is quite effective with children that are old enough to communicate their feelings. It gives your child the chance to talk to someone about the emotional side of ADHD. There is an emotional side to this disorder. Being unable to control his impulses, being hyperactive and always feeling "wired up," and dealing with the myriad of other ADHD symptoms are bound to take a toll on your child's feelings. Cognitive behavioral therapy will teach him how to look at himself in a positive and encouraging manner. It will help improve his self-esteem while helping him manage his behaviors. Used in conjunction with traditional behavior therapy, you and your child are likely to see great results.

PARENTAL THERAPY

This therapy is for you, the parent. This form of therapy should be used in conjunction as the behavior therapy your child receives. Think of parental therapy as a type of parent training course. Every parent has wished at one time or another that their child came with a parenting handbook. Well, therapy for parents is going to serve as that handbook. It will teach you how to cope with your child's different behaviors. It is your chance to talk about how his behaviors affect you. You will talk about how you handle his behaviors, such as yelling too much or not being consistent with your expectations and consequences. The therapist is going to teach you how to respond to ADHD behaviors. Remember, your responses mean a lot to your child. They affect how he feels because your reactions, especially if they are negative, could be telling him you might not like him.

During parental therapy, you will be given the tools that you need to manage your ADHD child's behaviors at home. Teaching you how to change your own parenting skills can be daunting and even a little insulting. However, you must keep an open mind because you cannot expect positive changes in your child without changing yourself for the better, too. Once you are equipped with the strategies and tools that you need to manage ADHD behaviors in a positive, encouraging manner, you will start to see the changes reflected in your child. He is going to notice when you are no longer yelling at him for not listening but gently reminding him instead. These types of changes are quite impactful on the feelings of an ADHD child.

SOCIAL SKILLS THERAPY

This type of therapy is more of a form of training for your ADHD child. It is especially useful if your child struggles in social settings. Learning and improving social skills will help your child to interact better with his peers. If your child is particularly antisocial, then social skills therapy will help him learn how to behave in a social environment. The environment may be at school, daycare, or just a playdate. The goal of social skills therapy is to arm your ADHD child with the tools and techniques he needs to behave in an acceptable and appropriate manner when interacting with other children or being in a public, social setting, such as at church or in a restaurant.

Basic social skills can include sharing, taking turns, and coping with teasing or hurtful words from a peer. Your ADHD child has to learn how to handle different types of social situations without having a meltdown or becoming aggressive. Older children might learn how to calm their anxiety in a crowded room. They may need skills in learning how to talk to peers, even just simple conversations, especially if the older child has social anxiety. Social skills therapy will provide your child with the tools that he can take with him even as he grows older. There will always be social settings—school, work, stores, concerts—and with social skills therapy, your ADHD child will know how to handle himself and his behaviors in all of those settings and many more.

FAMILY THERAPY

This is a type of therapy that is for the entire family. ADHD does not affect only the child; it affects the entire family. It is a disorder that is often disruptive to the family unit, as we discussed earlier. The goal of family therapy is to help each member of your family cope with ADHD behaviors. The behaviors of your child affect each person in a different way. Family therapy will address each member of the family in private and as a group. It will teach each family member how to deal with their own feelings about ADHD and how it has personally affected them.

This is an emotional form of talking therapy. Each session will give the entire family a chance to voice their feelings and concerns. Everyone is not expected to agree. Everyone is not expected to always react the right way to ADHD behaviors. Family therapy can be quite emotionally-charged. Each person's feelings are valid, even negative feelings. Each session gives the family the opportunity to talk to a neutral third-party. The therapist will listen to each concern, and she will aid the family in communicating with each other in constructive, positive ways.

BENEFITS OF THERAPY

Now that you have a better understanding of some of the

available therapy options, it is easier to see why some parents use therapy as the only form of ADHD treatment for their child. Therapy has numerous advantages in comparison to other methods of treatment.

- The biggest advantage is that your child does not have to take prescription drugs. Drugs always have the potential for side effects. With therapy, you do not have to worry about physical side effects.

- Therapy focuses on actually modifying the ADHD behaviors, while medication focuses on suppressing the behaviors. With therapy, your child will learn life skills for managing his behaviors.

- With so many options of therapy available, your ADHD child will receive help in all aspects of coping with his behaviors. From behavior modification to social skills, your child will be immersed in therapeutic treatment for his ADHD.

- The success rate of therapy as an ADHD treatment method is high. Adults and children have both had great success utilizing various forms of therapy to manage their ADHD behaviors for the long-term.

- Therapy will help you as the parent, as well as the rest of your child's family. Since ADHD is a disorder that affects the entire family unit, therapy is quite beneficial to everyone involved.

- If your ADHD child does need medication, the use of therapy at the same time will still be effective. Therapy can make it possible for your child to eventually not need the medications any longer because his behaviors have actually modified into something more manageable.

When you examine all of the advantages of therapy—and the above list is certainly not a complete list of advantages—it definitely becomes a potential option for treating ADHD. Therapy will help your child and the entire family unit to face ADHD and its problems as a team, a united front that is determined to defeat ADHD together.

POSSIBLE DISADVANTAGES OF THERAPY

Clearly, there are numerous types of therapy available to help manage your child's ADHD. Therapy is a positive, non-prescription method of treating the disorder. It can be successful as the sole form of treatment, and it can be successful when used with other methods of treatment including medication. However, as with anything, there can be some disadvantages associated with therapy. Just as you need to familiarize yourself with the potential side effects of medication, you also need to understand the possible disadvantages of therapeutic ADHD treatment.

- Probably the biggest disadvantage to therapy is that it is not going to give you instant results. One session is not going to have a noticeable impact on your child's ADHD behaviors. Therapy takes time and patience to make a difference in his ADHD. You may find yourself getting frustrated as a parent because you need these behaviors to change. Your ADHD child may also feel frustrated if he feels like he is not succeeding with therapy. These feelings of frustration will only make the ADHD behaviors worse.

- The therapist and your ADHD child may not "click." For any type of one-on-one therapy to be successful, there has to be trust and communication between the therapist and the patient. If your child does not feel comfortable talking to and working with the therapist, the therapy is not going to be successful. It may take a few different therapists before you find one that your ADHD child trusts.

- Your ADHD child simply may not be successful with

therapy. Therapists are not always successful in modifying behaviors. You and your child have to be willing to put in the work. If your ADHD child is not willing or able to work with you and the therapist on his behaviors, then therapy will not be successful. The same applies to you as the parent. If you are not willing to put in the work to help your child modify his behaviors at home, the therapy will not be successful.

- Family therapy can be emotionally exhausting and explosive. There is always a chance that someone in the family is going to be hurt by the words or actions of a family member during a session. Even though the therapist is trained to help your family get through the spectrum of emotions, it can still be difficult to handle, especially for your ADHD child and any siblings.

- Therapy can be quite expensive. Depending on your insurance or financial situation, therapy may not be an affordable option for treating your child's ADHD. It can cause a significant strain on the family finances, which can lead to strain on the family unit, including marriages.

While there are not many true disadvantages related to therapy, you do need to weigh the pros and cons of therapy for your ADHD child. You also have to decide what type of therapy you want for him, as well as if you are willing to utilize therapy for yourself and your family. You still have a family to consider in addition to your ADHD child, so you have to ensure that you can afford the therapy sessions. If you decide that therapy is the best option, your child's doctor can provide you with the names of therapists specializing in ADHD treatment.

Professional help, like the different therapy options, is ideal for helping your child learn to manage his ADHD. It is even helpful to you, the parent because you will be given tools and strategies to use, as well. As a team, you, your child, and the therapist will work together to modify his behaviors, rather than just suppress them with medications. All of this is very helpful in the big picture. But, what about the smaller picture? What about the regular, everyday life that you and your ADHD child have to live? How do you live with an ADHD child without having to be in constant therapy mode? It really is not as difficult as you might think.

CHAPTER 7:

METHODS FOR LIVING WITH AN ADHD CHILD

By this point, you have taken in a lot of ADHD information. You know what it is and all of the available treatment options for your child. You now know that he does not have to suffer from ADHD in vain. The disorder can be managed—your child will be able to live with ADHD. While you have also learned of the available help to you as the parent of an ADHD child, the day-to-day life can be difficult. Knowing how to live with an ADHD child is vital to the success of treating his disorder, and it will make life that much easier for you as his parent. There are various methods that you can use at home to aid in ADHD treatment.

PARENTAL TIPS AND TOOLS

Being the parent of an ADHD child requires patience and understanding more than anything else. Your child is certain to push you to your limits on different occasions. The various ADHD behaviors can be frustrating for you. There are numerous ways that you can make life at home better for your child and the family. Behavior management goes beyond the therapy sessions with your ADHD child. Managing the behaviors at home can be tough, but it is definitely doable. These tips and tools will help you manage and cope with ADHD at home.

- **Acceptance** – You have to accept that your child has ADHD. This means that he is not exactly like other children or even his siblings. Acceptance is essential to your child because he needs to know that he is loved, no matter what. It can be tough for a parent to believe that their child has a disorder. However, the quicker you accept the diagnosis, the faster you can start modifying behaviors with your child.

- **Rules** – At home, you have to clearly define the rules. With an ADHD child, you cannot simply say that running is not allowed. Words are likely to go in one ear and out the other. Your child needs clear, precise rules for the home. The best thing to do is to write them down and display the rules in a prominent place in the house. Your child will have a visual aid to remind him of the rules at all times.

- **Be consistent** – As mentioned earlier, consistency is the key to modifying behaviors. It is imperative that you follow through on both rewards and consequences. ADHD children need consistency in their lives. They need to know that when a parent says something, it will happen. Failing to follow through is only going to make your ADHD child not trust your word. He is more likely to push those boundaries to see how far he can go.

- **Routines** – ADHD children thrive with routine schedules. You must establish a routine for your child that you can both adhere to every day. The daily routines do not necessarily have to be the same. For instance, weekday routines and weekend routines can differ. The important thing is that you follow these routines every day and every week. Routines become habits, and you want your ADHD child to establish good habits. Prepare a written schedule your child can look at whenever he needs a reminder about what he should be doing or what is coming.

- **Immediate rewards and consequences** – When managing ADHD at home, you have to give an immediate response to your child's behaviors. You cannot wait to give him a consequence because he may not even remember what happened later. The same is true for rewards. He needs to know right away when he does something positive or something negative. The immediate reactions will begin to mold his behaviors at home.

- **Be positive** – As a parent, you need to look at each and every situation with a positive attitude. Even bad situations should be dealt with in a supportive manner. Your ADHD child needs encouragement for even the little things. Positivity will help your child have a better self-esteem and build confidence. Just make sure that you are not putting too much pressure on your child by being positive about everything. You can be supportive of him when he has a behavioral mishap without making him feel like it is okay to behave in a negative manner.

- **Be flexible** – Yes, your child needs rules and structure and routine. He will thrive with a schedule. However, this is an ADHD child you are living with, and you simply must allow room for flexibility. There is no guarantee that every rule or routine will always be followed without problems. Prepare for the unexpected so that when it happens, you are ready. There are going to be lots of times when your child will need gentle reminders before you start handing out consequences. Remember: you are not perfect, and you should not expect perfection from your ADHD child.

- **Stay Organized** – Lack of organization will only slow down your child's progress. He is easily distracted and forgetful. Therefore, he needs his living space organized in a way that enhances his life. One thing you can do is organize his bedroom. Use baskets with labels to make sure he knows where all of his things belong. Create a quiet place for homework that is free from distractions. Think of it like this: your ADHD child's mind is already in an almost constant state of disarray and disorder. A peaceful, organized environment at home can help calm is mind.

- **Cut down on screen time** – Children enjoy gaming and television. While it is not necessary to completely cut off screen time, you do need to control it. Encourage activities outside. Play board games with the family. Try to keep your child active and engaged to prevent boredom. Do not let the PS4 or cable television become a babysitter for your child. Sure, it might give you a few moments of peace, but is it really helping your ADHD child? Consider using screen time as a part of positive reinforcement. For example, your child can earn extra time on his favorite video game by achieving weekly goals.

- **Interaction** – Another vital tool for living with an ADHD child is to interact with him. Talk to your child. Listen to his thoughts and ideas. Ask him about his day at school. Let your child know that you are interested in his life. This is also a chance for you to encourage waiting for his turn to speak because the two of you are having a conversation. No child, with ADHD or not, likes to feel ignored by their loved ones. Make time every day to interact one-on-one with your child.

- **Sleep routines** – So many ADHD children have trouble sleeping. Since sleep is the body's way of healing and recharging for the next day, it is obvious why it is so important. Create a nightly routine that will help your child relax, fall asleep, and stay asleep. Sleep sounds playing in the background can be helpful. A calming lavender bath before bedtime is relaxing. Follow the routine each night to help your child establish a sleep pattern that lets him get the rest that he needs.

- **Learn how to say yes** – It is easy for all parents to fall into the habit of always saying no to a child's request. Make the effort to start saying yes to reasonable requests. If your ADHD child always hears you telling him no, he is more likely to rebel against you. Listen to your child's requests and pay attention. For instance, is a late-night snack really going to cause some sort of problem for your child? Even when you have to say no, talk about your decision with your child. Explain why you are saying no instead of just expecting him to accept it.

- **Be prepared** – Do not expect your child to behave all of the time. It simply is not going to happen, especially with an ADHD child. This is true in and out of the house. Before you and your child go to the store or visit a friend, sit him down and make a plan. Discuss your expectations for his behavior during the outing and discuss the consequences and rewards. Your ADHD child always needs to know what he can expect. Learn to see the signs of when your child is about to have a meltdown. It is always easier to stop it before it gets started.

TAKING CARE OF THE PARENT

All of this time, we have focused on what you can do for your ADHD child. But you are only human. You have to incorporate self-care into your life, too. Living with an ADHD child is not easy. You are going to be pushed to your limits. You are going to feel overwhelmed and frustrated. You are likely to lose your temper. Just as you need to know when your child is about to lose control, you must recognize those signs within yourself. The following tips will help you take the best care of yourself so that you can take the best care of your child.

- Take a break when you feel yourself reaching your limits. This is essentially giving yourself a time-out. Parents get stressed and overwhelmed, too, especially when dealing with ADHD. Do not let ADHD control every aspect of your life. Instead, walk away from a tough situation and give yourself time to calm down. When you are calm, you can return to the situation with a clear head and better determine how to handle it.

- To get calm, try meditation or even the "count to ten" method. Deep breathing and other relaxation techniques will help you get back in control of your own emotions.

Remember that your ADHD child is watching you. He needs to see that even you, the parent, gets frustrated. He needs to see how you deal with the emotions, and he can even learn how to calm himself with you. Come up with a code word that basically puts the situation or argument on hold while the two of you get centered and refocused. If he is on the verge of an outburst, and you can feel your nerves reaching their limit, use the code word to signal hitting the pause button while both of you use relaxation and calming techniques to regain control of emotions. Then, both of you will come back to the scenario with a calm, clear mind.

- Ask for help when you need it. You need time for yourself. Do not be afraid to make that time for yourself by enlisting in the help of your family or even a babysitter. As long as everyone understands the needs of your ADHD child, there is nothing wrong with letting someone else take over for a little while. This gives you the chance to get out and recharge. Go to the gym or just take a walk. Go to the movies or treat yourself to a manicure and pedicure.

- Utilize therapy options for yourself. Talking over ADHD issues with a professional can be quite helpful in reducing stress. A professional can give you proven advice and techniques to use at home. Even venting to a friend can help. While your friend may not have useful advice for you, getting things off of your chest can be a very good stress reliever. You do not need to keep your own thoughts and feelings bottled up inside. Find a safe environment to let them out.

A happy, healthy parent is vital to the overall treatment of ADHD and living with the accompanying behaviors. Take care of yourself when you need it. Make time every week just for you. Go ahead and take that long bubble bath. The better you are, the better your child is likely to be.

DISCIPLINING THE ADHD CHILD

As you get closer to being practically a master of ADHD, there is one aspect of the disorder that we have not thoroughly discussed—discipline. An extremely important part of raising children, regardless of ADHD, is discipline. Children need a form of discipline to learn that there are consequences for unacceptable behaviors. They need the boundaries and rules that come with discipline. From the time they are toddlers to when they are young adults, children are constantly discovering their boundaries. When they push the limits of those boundaries, that is when it becomes necessary to discipline them. Your ADHD child is no exception. As with all children, there is a right and wrong way to provide discipline. The following tips will help you to ensure that you are disciplining the right way.

- **Know the difference between discipline and punishment** – Punishment, like spanking, yelling, grounding, taking away toys, is a way to force your ADHD child to behave the way that you want. Discipline focuses on actually teaching your child how to behave without fear or shame. You need your child to understand why a consequence is happening, rather than just having him fear the punishment. He will take what he learns with him when he is an adult. Teach him about correcting his behavior instead of trying to force him out of fear.

- **Remember the disorder** – Before handing out a consequence as a form of discipline, remember that your child has ADHD. There are simply some behaviors that he may not be able to control. Getting distracted easily is a big factor in the life of an ADHD child. He does not mean to stop doing his chores—he just gets distracted by other, more interesting things. Sometimes, the best thing you can do is just remind your child of what he should be doing. Not everything requires a consequence.

- **Time-out** – Time-outs are a useful tool in disciplining an ADHD child. When a situation is going south quickly, simply remove your child from the situation and place him in a time-out. Sure, he might resist, especially if he is already in the middle of an outburst or temper tantrum, but the time-out gives him a chance to calm down and collect himself. Sometimes, the problem is overstimulation. A time-out removes your child from the excess stimulation so that he can settle down and try again.

- **Do not label your child** – Telling your ADHD child he is lazy because he did not do his chores, or he is a pig because his room is a mess is not acceptable. You are the parent. You cannot label your child with these types of hurtful words because it is damaging to his self-esteem. Think before you speak. Ask yourself if you would want to be labeled in a negative way. Then, find a positive way to approach the situation without using labels that stick to your ADHD child.

- **Ignore** – There are certain behaviors that you need to just ignore. These can include things like whining, repeatedly asking you for something when you have already said no, and general complaining. Children seek attention. Even negative attention is better than no attention at all. This is especially true of ADHD children. When you ignore mild behaviors that are simply your child being annoying or obnoxious, he will learn that those kinds of behaviors do not get him any attention. It has to be reiterated—not every behavior requires a consequence.

- **Choose your battles** – This disciplining tip is true for all children, not just ADHD children. Some things are not worth fighting over. It is okay to let minor things slide now and then. It is also okay to let your child make a choice for himself that may not be the best choice. For example, if your child refuses to eat dinner, do not be afraid to let him miss a meal. If he decides right before bed that he is hungry, it is too late. He made his choice. It is not going to kill him, and he will eventually learn that he needs to eat when it is time for dinner.

- **Keep grounding reasonable** – This is especially important for older ADHD children. When you ground your child, make it specific. He needs to know when the grounding will end because he needs to know that there is an end in sight. If you constantly add to his grounding, or you are vague in the length of the grounding, he may just stop caring at all. He might do whatever he wants anyway because he is already grounded, and he does not know when it will end.

- **Think before you discipline** – Try not to react out of frustration or anger when you are disciplining your ADHD child. You may overreact and feel guilty later. If you do overreact while disciplining, take the time to explain and apologize to your child. He needs to know that parents make mistakes, too.

These are just a few methods to aid you in disciplining your ADHD child. It is important that you do not use the disorder as a constant excuse for your child's behavior. You also cannot allow him to use ADHD as an excuse. It is acceptable to have behavior expectations for your child the same way you expect good behavior from a non-ADHD child. It may take a little more time and effort to get the right behavior out of your child, but he can learn to behave. When the situation calls for discipline, think it through and apply the appropriate consequence.

ADHD ACTIVITIES FOR THE CHILD

With all of this talk about managing behaviors and discipline, it is no surprise if you feel like ADHD is going to be almost like a job for you to handle. While it can be hard to live with an ADHD child, there are a number of things you can do with your child or encourage him to do on his own to keep him busy and out of trouble. ADHD children have lots of pent-up energy and creativity. These activities could be a great outlet for your child to burn off energy and let his creative juices flow!

- **Board games** – Who remembers the thrill of playing Monopoly as a child? Heck, even adults love the real estate buying and selling game. Board games are a great activity for your ADHD child because they give him something to focus on that is fun and entertaining. Start off with simple board games, like Trouble or Sorry, because you do not want your child to get bored or lose interest. Board games can also teach him patience and taking turns, and how to be a good sport if he loses!

- **Scouts** – Consider signing your ADHD child up for a scout program. These programs have been around for a long time. They teach children all kinds of skills, and they have a lot of fun competitions, such as push-car races. Scouts already use a reward system of badges that will encourage your child to achieve his goal and master the skill they are working on.

- **Children's theater** – This is also a great way to keep your child engaged and active. Your ADHD child might enjoy acting out a play in a theater setting geared towards kids. Not only does it give him a big responsibility of learning his lines, it also gives him a chance to pretend and role-play.

- **Tell stories** – If you need a simple activity for your child, sit down and tell stories. Make it a game. You can start the story with a sentence or two and then your child can add to the story. This is a good way to let his imagination take charge. You can also take turns telling stories to each other. See who can come up with the best story of the day.

- **Music** – Another good activity for ADHD children is music, both singing and playing an instrument. Studies have already proven the positive effects music programs have on children in school. Bring those positive effects home by having karaoke contests in the living room. You can even form a band together and use household items for instruments. Take it a step further, and invest in some yard-sale instruments that your child can play with at home.

- **Go outside** – Playing outside is always a great choice for the active ADHD child. Biking, running, swimming, playing tag, and hide and seek are all options for outdoor activities. Your child is full of energy, so if he has the chance to burn some of it off outside, let him. Make it a family activity and join in on the fun.

- **Scavenger hunt** – A scavenger hunt is a fun game to play inside the house where you can keep a watchful eye on your ADHD child. On a rainy day, get a few items, hide them around the house, and write down clues for your child. Then, help him solve the clues and find the items. Think of a fun reward you can give him for collecting all the items.

- **Charades** – Charades is another imagination outlet. Letting your child act out different words lets him use his creativity to make you guess the answer. It is also a good chance for helping him build his reading skills and even learn new words. Involve the whole family in a night of charades for some good, wholesome fun.

- **Just dance** – Dancing is a fun way to get some exercise and have a great time doing it. Put on your child's favorite music and have an impromptu dance party at home. Get crazy, and let your dancing skills shine, too. You can even make a game out of it. For instance, every time the music stops, everyone has to freeze. The last person standing gets a prize.

- **Arts and crafts** – These are classic activities that all children enjoy. Your ADHD child is sure to love making slime, painting with his fingers or brushes, or weaving on a child's plastic loom. This is your child's chance to really be creative, and who knows? You just might have the next Picasso living in your home.

It is plain to see that there are plenty of methods to make living with an ADHD child easier. ADHD is a tough disorder to manage—you need patience, determination, and even professional assistance. However, the point is that ADHD is manageable. Life at home does not have to be a constant battle or challenge. Utilize the tips and ideas given to you here, as well as discover your own. The internet is an awesome resource for finding answers to your questions or getting ideas for activities. Life with an ADHD child is still just life with a child. Enjoy it. Make the most of it. ADHD is not going to destroy your child's ability to have a normal life.

CHAPTER 8:

LOOKING ON THE BRIGHT SIDE OF ADHD

Throughout this book, we have discussed all aspects of ADHD—understanding what ADHD is, the symptoms and possible associated conditions, when and how to get a diagnosis, ADHD treatments, therapy and counseling, and methods for living with ADHD. While every bit of this information is useful because knowledge is power, there is one thing we have yet to discuss—the bright side of ADHD. You are probably reading this and thinking about all the negative behavioral and emotional issues. You are probably wondering how it is possible to be optimistic about a neurobiological disorder, especially one that is affecting the lives of your child and your family. But ADHD is not a prison sentence defined as life with no chance of parole. It is not a prison at all, especially when you change the way you view the disorder. Now, it is time to examine the good parts of ADHD.

THE POSITIVE SIDE OF ADHD

The first step in examining the positive side of ADHD is to transform your perspective. Stop looking at it from a negative viewpoint. Stop dwelling on the bad side of the behavioral issues, and start looking at them as beneficial personality attributes. For each negative behavioral trait, there is an opposite—a "mirror" trait that ignores the negativity and focuses solely on the positive. Below is a list of some of the negative ADHD attributes and their corresponding "mirror" traits. As you can see, it is all about perspective and how you choose to view each behavior.

- Impulsive behavior – Creative energy

- Moody and irritable – Sensitive and compassionate

- Easily distracted – Curious about the world around them

- Restless and hyperactive – Energetic and ready for adventure

- Stubborn – Determined

- Pushy and forward – Enthusiastic and assertive

When you focus on the "mirror" qualities of your child's behavior, you discover an entirely new way of living. You no longer have to cope with the disruptive behaviors. Instead, you and your ADHD child can find new avenues to explore by using his "mirror" traits. There will still be times when those negative behaviors rear their ugly heads. But now you have the knowledge and skill set to deal with the negative behaviors swiftly, turning a potentially heated encounter into a positive situation.

In addition to finding the "mirror" qualities of your ADHD child, there are other positives to having ADHD. The ADHD mind might come across as unfocused and distractible, constantly leaping from one thought to another. However, this particular quality can come in quite handy for solving problems. As the mind of your ADHD child examines a problem with a peer, he is likely to sort through solutions faster than the non-ADHD child. While the non-ADHD child is still evaluating the first or second possible solution, your child has probably evaluated all of the solutions and may even be ready to solve the problem. ADHD children observe so many small details around them as they try to take in everything they see and hear. Your ADHD child is probably hearing much more than you realize. Just because your child appears to be involved in a different activity does not mean he is not also paying attention to your conversation. So, you may want to think twice before discussing adult matters in front of him.

Even though your ADHD child might have to work twice as hard as others, this is not necessarily a type of handicap. Instead, knowing that goals do not come as easily to him often intensifies the resolve of your ADHD child. His increased sense of determination pushes him to try and try again until he reaches his goal. Having this sort of determination may come across at times as stubbornness, but when you look at the "mirror" quality, you and your child will realize that persevering can be quite fulfilling. ADHD children are also not always unfocused. When they find an activity or task that excites them and keeps them intrigued, they can actually become intensely focused. This intense focus is so captivating that they often forget the entire world around them. Focusing like this can be quite helpful in completing projects, reading books, and overall learning.

Another positive side of ADHD is the seemingly endless amount of energy within your child. This type of infinite energy is useful in extracurricular activities, such as sports. Your ADHD child will probably want to participate in as many activities as possible. Baseball, football, and track are good examples for burning off that energy supply. While you may be concerned with injuries or worried that your child might fail, his thoughts are somewhere else. He is not as likely to be afraid of failure because learning to live with ADHD has taught him to persevere and push forward, no matter what. Even taking a family hike in the hills will be an adventure for your ADHD child. Not only does your child expend some extra energy, but he also gets the chance to spend time with his family. All of this physical activity not only keeps boredom at bay, but it is also good for your child's physical health.

Another encouraging aspect of ADHD is your child's ability to be compassionate and accepting of others. What someone might see as overly emotional is just your child being deeply in tune with his emotions and being unable to hold them inside. Sure, this can be trying at times, but in times of crisis, such as when a loved one passes away, you can almost bet that your ADHD child will be a great source of comfort. Compassion comes easily to your ADHD child. He understands and connects with emotions. In fact, ADHD children are often described as having the biggest hearts and sensitive souls. It is not uncommon to find your child crying during emotional movies because of his enhanced sense of compassion.

Your ADHD child is also likely to have a very accepting personality. It will not matter if a potential friend seems "different" than everyone else. This is because your ADHD child is already special himself, so he understands what the other child is feeling. Your ADHD child does not care if a peer is the "underdog." A friend is a friend, and your child will enjoy having a new companion to play with and share creative energy. ADHD children have big personalities to match their big hearts. They make friends easily because they have such an interest in the world and what is happening around them. They have a zest for life that draws others' attention to them like moths to a flame.

One very important "mirror" trait is creativity. Your ADHD child is full of thoughts and ideas that need an outlet. His imagination is running wild at all hours of the day and night. Help your child to harness that creativity in a constructive way. Give your child a sketchbook or notebook so that he has a place to write down his thoughts and ideas, a place to draw the images that never seem to stop playing in his mind. You never know—maybe he will become the next big inventor! At the very least, the two of you can have interesting conversations about his thoughts and ideas. It is also a good idea if you embrace your ADHD child's imagination. Go ahead, get on the floor and play with your child. Maybe it is with Legos, maybe it is with a race track, and maybe it is just the two of you pretending to be characters in a fantasy land. Let your child's wild imagination help you release the kid inside.

ADHD can be difficult to deal with every day. There is no doubt that the constant struggle to modify and cope with behaviors is hard on your ADHD child, as well as the rest of the family. However, keeping things in perspective—especially a positive perspective—will help make each day just a little bit easier. This positive outlook will also rub off onto your ADHD child, encouraging him to embrace his differences and live his very best life for the rest of his life.

LIVING A NORMAL LIFE WITH ADHD

One of your primary concerns as a parent is probably how to maintain a normal life for your ADHD child, as well as for the rest of your family unit. All parents want well-behaved children that grow up to be contributing members of society. You may wonder if ADHD is going to hold your child back from reaching his full potential. Disruptive behaviors are also going to wear on your nerves, along with your family's nerves. There may be times when you find yourself wishing that your child could just be "normal." But your child is normal. He may not be like the average child, but he is normal. What you mean is that you wish your child did not have ADHD disrupting his life. You simply cannot dwell on the way things might have been—ADHD is a part of your lives now.

When talking about living a normal life with an ADHD child, you must think about the meaning of normal. One person's normal is another person's chaos. Just as you have to turn negative behaviors into positive "mirror" attributes, you need a positive outlook on life if you expect any sense of normalcy. Ask yourself what it means to you to have a normal life. Then, ask your ADHD child what it means to him. Compare your answers and you might just be surprised. A normal life for your family unit is not going to be like any other family. This is simply because values vary—what is important to one person may not be important to another. Just like that famous movie says, "Stupid is as stupid does." The same applies to normal. Your normal life may not look like everyone else's— but it is normal for you and your family—that is what really counts in the big picture. No one else is living your life for you, so no one else has the right to tell you what is and is not normal.

One important thing to remember in the long run is that even with an ADHD diagnosis, your life and the life of your child is only going to get better. No longer will you throw your hands up in the air and wonder why he is behaving in such a manner. No longer will you have to worry and wonder about what other parents think about your child and how they judge your parenting skills. With an ADHD diagnosis, you now know why. You also have the skills to properly handle every situation, even the bad ones. Being professionally diagnosed with ADHD is your child's first step to a better and more normal life. From that point on, between treatment and therapy, your child's behaviors are only going to improve. It may not be easy, but once you and your ADHD child have discovered what works best for him, life will be much easier on both of you.

The answers to a normal life may or may not lie in medications and therapy. You and your ADHD child must find the best solution for his particular situation. Remember, no two ADHD children are alike. They may display some of the same behaviors, but every person is unique. What works best for your friend's child may not even touch your child's behaviors. A key factor in your child living a normal life with ADHD is to stay consistent with the treatment plan. Even if his behaviors improve with age, do not stop treatment without warning. Instead, redefine the plan. Come up with something new. As your ADHD child gets older, he may not need medication or counseling three times a week. A simple group therapy session a few times a month might be enough. Again, the goal is to do what is best for your ADHD child's personal situation.

As your child grows up into an ADHD adult, assuming that his symptoms do not subside, treatment is still important. The level needed depends on the changing behaviors. Your goal as a parent is to see your child succeed in life. Whether that success comes from being a fry-cook or from being a senator, as long as your adult child is content and has the ability to function daily, you have done your job as a parent. Even in the event that your adult child winds up suffering from severe ADHD and associated conditions, requiring him to live at home or in a controlled environment, he can still have a normal life. The definition of a normal life merely changes to fit the new parameters. There simply is no reason why an ADHD child or an ADHD adult cannot live a normal life. Rather than focusing on the normalcy or the idea of normalcy, focus instead on joy and happiness. Does it really matter what anyone else thinks as long as your ADHD child/adult child is happy?

Remember the risk-taking that was discussed in earlier chapters? In the right environment, not being afraid of taking risks is beneficial to your ADHD child. Maybe he will have the courage to go ahead and try out for the school play, something you were always too shy to do when you were young. Taking risks can come in handy, especially as your ADHD child grows into adulthood. Maybe his love for science will lead him to take a chance in the lab and make new discoveries. Taking chances is a part of life, and the ADHD adult embraces the challenges. As mentioned earlier, there is a dangerous side to taking risks. However, diligent and proactive parents such as yourself can help teach their ADHD child how to evaluate situations before plunging in head first and your child will carry this information with him into adulthood. So, hopefully, you will not have to worry about dangerous risk-taking behaviors, only the fun and beneficial ones.

Another positive aspect of adult ADHD is his ability to stay calm during times of crisis. Studies have shown that the ADHD brain has more theta waves. These brain waves put the brain into what is known as "sleep mode." During a crisis, a non-ADHD person's brain becomes overloaded with the situation. Think of it as a circuit box that is overloaded and tripping breakers. A non-ADHD person is more likely to panic and not know what to do. However, an ADHD person's brain wakes up, right into what most consider a normal, functioning mode, rather than the sleep mode. So, while the other person panics and frantically runs around, confused and dazed, your adult child will find it easier to remain calm and rational. All because his brain is not overloaded with alarm, instead, it is actually functioning at its most normal level.

Another thing to keep in mind when evaluating the normalcy of your ADHD child's life is that his "mirror" qualities will still exist when he reaches adulthood. Even if the negative behaviors subside, your child can still embrace the positive "mirrors." Just because the ADHD adult no longer feels moody and irritable does not mean that he has to sacrifice being compassionate. Being in touch with your emotions is a good thing, even if you do not have ADHD or if your symptoms have subsided. When symptoms fail to subside as your child grows up, those "mirror" traits come in handy again. ADHD adults are often great at multitasking because their busy minds are able to keep up with all of the tasks at once—as long as the tasks are interesting. The ability to multitask is likely to help your adult child once he hits the job market. At the very least, you can expect your adult ADHD child to choose a line of work that keeps him busy and offers a variety of tasks to complete. Monotony will never be a friend to a child or an adult who has ADHD.

Back to the ADHD child, the best thing you can do as a parent is to let your child be a child. Embrace everything about him, including the ADHD. Your child did not ask for the disorder. Neither did you, of course. However, as the adult, it is your responsibility to provide a nurturing, patient, and loving environment for your child. Focus on the positive side of ADHD, the "mirrors" of each behavior. Teach your child to keep his eyes on the bright side. Let your positive thinking and energy rub off onto him so that he will carry that same positivity and energy throughout the rest of his days. Live life one day at a time, one situation at a time, and choose your battles with care. Millions of families all over the world live with ADHD within their midst. A positive outlook will be your family's strongest weapon in dealing with this condition and all that comes with it.

If you find yourself or your ADHD child or other family members still struggling day-to-day, never be afraid or embarrassed to reach out for help. In addition to your child's personal physician, there are countless therapy groups, internet forums, and even

Facebook groups and pages where all of you can find support and understanding. None of you have to face life with ADHD alone. Talking about the situations with strangers or a therapist helps by giving you a neutral perspective. It is also helpful to speak to people that live with ADHD in their family unit, too. They fully understand what each of you is going through, and they may even have helpful suggestions. Even during the toughest times, even when it does not seem like your life or the lives of your ADHD child and family could possibly be normal, remind yourself of one thing—it is just a bad day, it is not a bad life.

Yes, it is possible to live a completely normal life with ADHD. From childhood through adulthood, with treatment and by focusing on the advantages of ADHD, your child has a bright future. Even though approximately 50% of ADHD children continue to exhibit signs of ADHD into adulthood, that still means that the other 50% either seem to "grow out" of the disorder, or they have learned enough coping skills to be well-adjusted adults. Fifty-fifty odds are pretty good when it comes to ADHD. Just because your child may have difficulties with ADHD now does not mean he will always face these obstacles. Even if he does struggle with ADHD for the rest of his life, it can still be managed, and he can still live a full life. With the right treatment approach, focused therapy that teaches behavioral management and coping skills, and a supportive family unit behind him, your child will have his normal life.

CONCLUSION

Thank you for making it through to the end of *ADHD: Help Your Kids Reach Their Full Potential and Become Self-Regulated, Focused, and Confident*. Let's hope it was informative and able to provide you with all of the tools you need to achieve your goals whatever they may be.

ADHD, although a common condition, can be quite serious. There are so many symptoms that can affect your child's ability to live a happy life, as well as numerous other conditions that could interfere with his quality of living. Your child is lucky to have a parent in his life that is willing to go the extra mile, and educate yourself so thoroughly about ADHD.

The next step is to take your newfound ADHD information and start incorporating the tips, tools, and techniques revealed in this book into the life of your child. Knowledge is power, and this is especially true when dealing with a neurobehavioral disorder like ADHD. The effects ADHD can have on your child's brain and behaviors are absolutely astounding! You now know how ADHD affects your family and your child's education. You also know how to minimize those effects through different forms of treatment. From prescription medications to behavior modification therapy, and even dietary and lifestyle changes, you understand the many ways that ADHD can be managed with your child's well-being always coming first.

We all know that an ADHD diagnosis can be a scary thing to even think about, much less actually manage. But now you know that ADHD is not the end of the world for your child—with the right treatment and a supportive, loving environment, he will live his best life. The world is truly your child's oyster, even if he has to share it with ADHD. You, as a parent, have taken the right step by diving headfirst into the dizzying reality of ADHD. Keep your head up, stay positive, and take things one day at a time—even one tiny step at a time. It will not be long before the strategies you learned from this book will start to show results at home. While you may be in a bit of information overload right now, you will soon be grabbing ADHD right by the horns and helping your child show it who the boss is!

Finally, if you found this book useful in any way, a review on Amazon is always appreciated!

Best Regards,
Bill Andrews

More books by Bill Andrews
https://geni.us/billbooks

FREE BONUS
INTERVIEW WITH AN ADHD EXPERT

Thank you for downloading this book. As a way of showing my appreciation, I want to give you a **FREE BONUS interview** with an ADHD expert along with this book.

Has Your Child Been Diagnosed With ADHD? Is Coping With Your Child's Behavior Wearing You Out? Are You Tired of Searching For Answers?

If you answered yes, don't miss this BONUS interview with ADHD expert, Deena Kotlewski, MA, LCPC.

Inside You'll Learn...

- What are the three different types of ADHD?
- What are the biggest symptoms you should be on the lookout for?
- What causes ADHD?
- How should ADHD be treated?
- Learn about these little known secrets for coping with ADHD.
- ...and much, much more!

Go to the below URL for Instant Access
http://bit.ly/ADHDExpertInterview

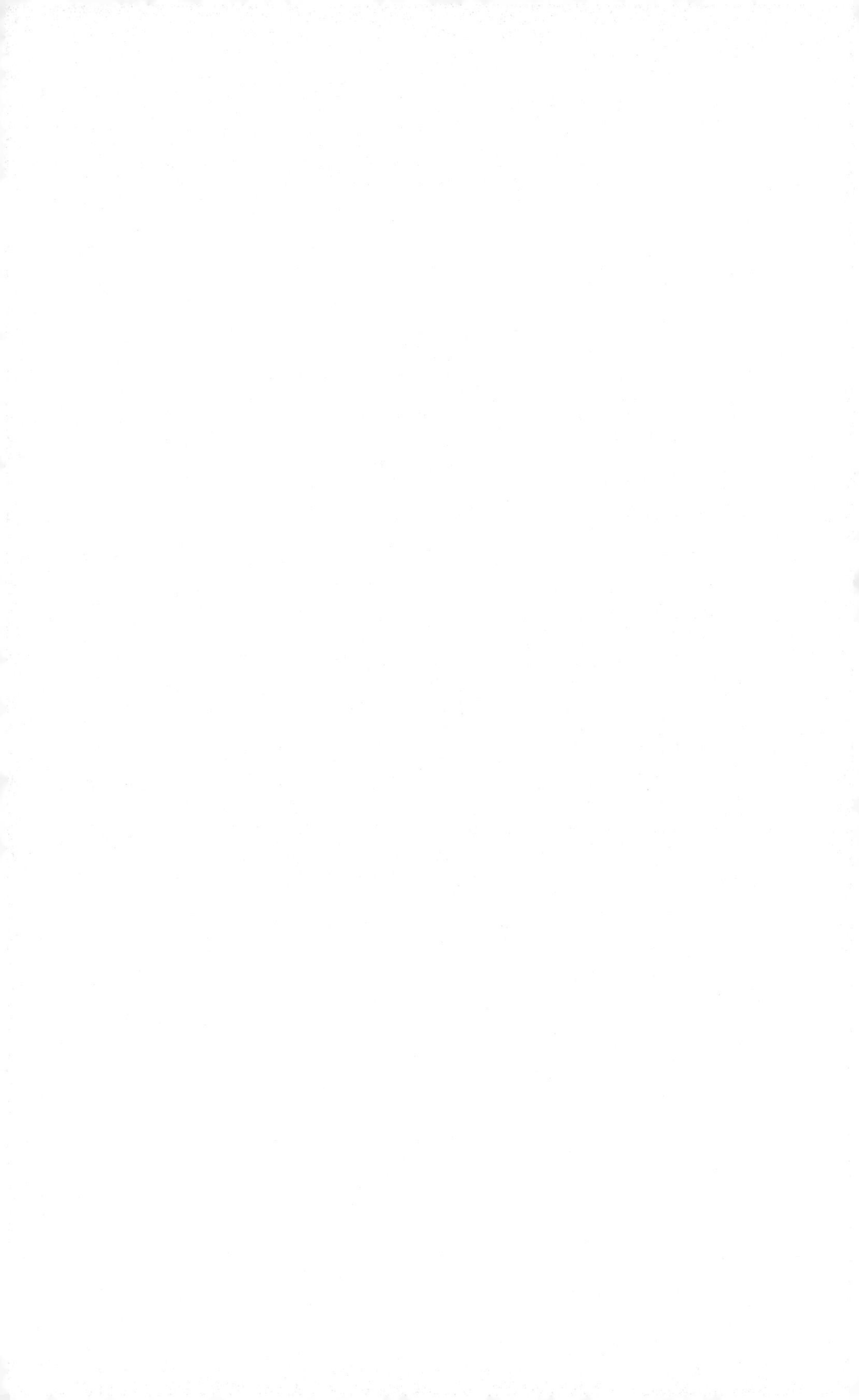

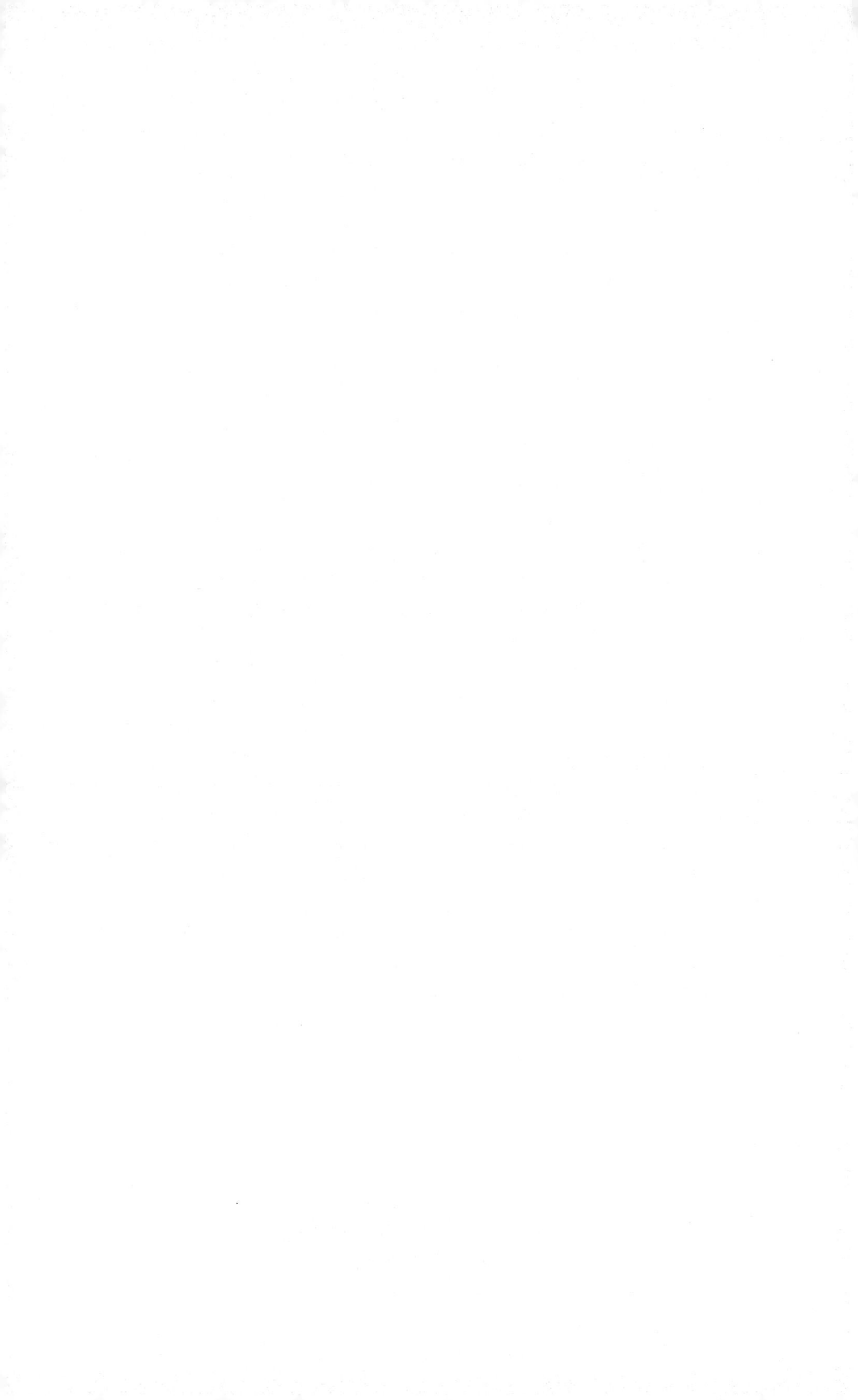

Made in the USA
Las Vegas, NV
01 December 2021